THE
HEALTHY
COCONUT

JENNI MADISON

ROCKPOOL
PUBLISHING

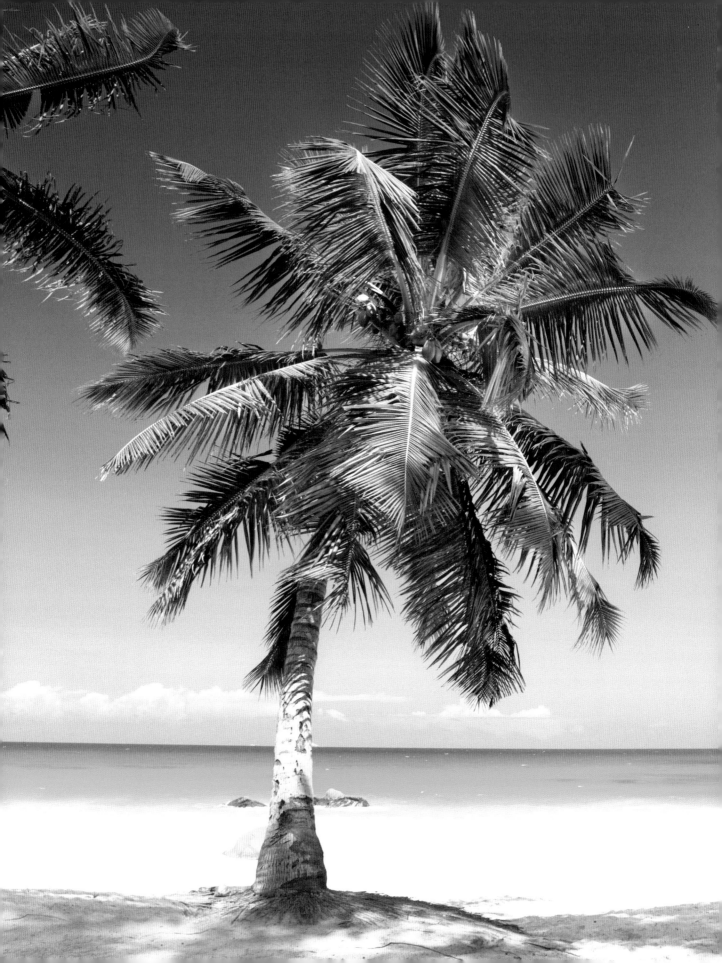

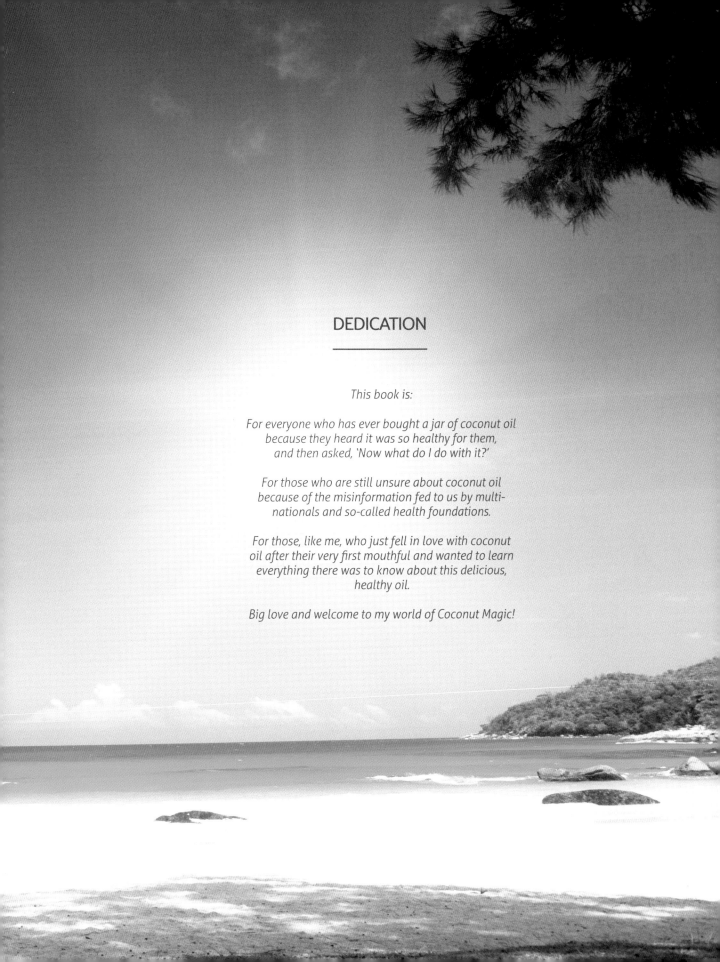

DEDICATION

_____

This book is:

*For everyone who has ever bought a jar of coconut oil
because they heard it was so healthy for them,
and then asked, 'Now what do I do with it?'*

*For those who are still unsure about coconut oil
because of the misinformation fed to us by multi-
nationals and so-called health foundations.*

*For those, like me, who just fell in love with coconut
oil after their very first mouthful and wanted to learn
everything there was to know about this delicious,
healthy oil.*

Big love and welcome to my world of Coconut Magic!

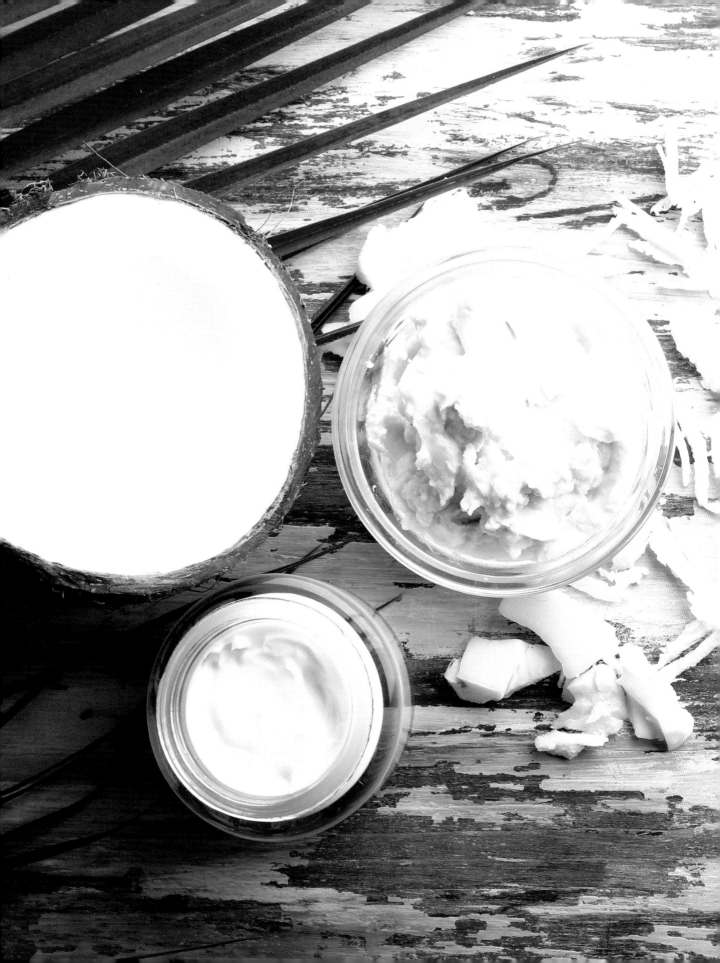

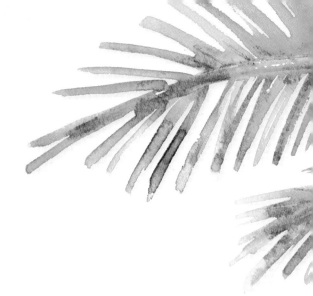

CONTENTS

Introduction 9

The Healthy Coconut.............................. 12

Healthy Oil Vs Toxic Oil 16

Types Of Fats.. 19

Natural Sugars Vs Processed Sugars................... 24

Low-Down On Sugars............................ 26

Choosing Your Coconut Oil................... 27

Nutritive Benefits Of Virgin Coconut Oil.......... 34

How To Use Coconut Oil........................ 35

Diet And Lifestyle Choices.................... 36

Coconut Oil For Detox And Energy 46

Healthy Fats For Healthy Weight.......... 47

Coconut Oil And Coconut For Health 48

Brain Health 49

Pregnancy And Baby Care 53

Hormone And Thyroid Health 54

The Candida Cleanse.............................. 56

Oil Pulling Therapy 58

Coconut Oil For Healing 60

Coconut Oil For Beauty.......................... 62

Coconut Oil And Sex.............................. 67

Coconut Oil And Healthy Pets.............. 69

What The Experts Are Saying 70

THE HEALTHY COCONUT RECIPES

Smoothies, Juices & Teas 72

Breakfast 88

Plant-Based Butter, Milk, Cheese,
Cream & Yoghurt....................................106

Soups 116

Main Meals 130

Snacks, Sides & Dips 156

Super Salads & Salad Dressings 166

Raw Chocolate.......................................184

Healthy Desserts....................................202

Coconut Body Care & Beauty 220

Glossary Of Products............................228

Index 232

Acknowledgements 240

About The Author...................................241

Publishing...242

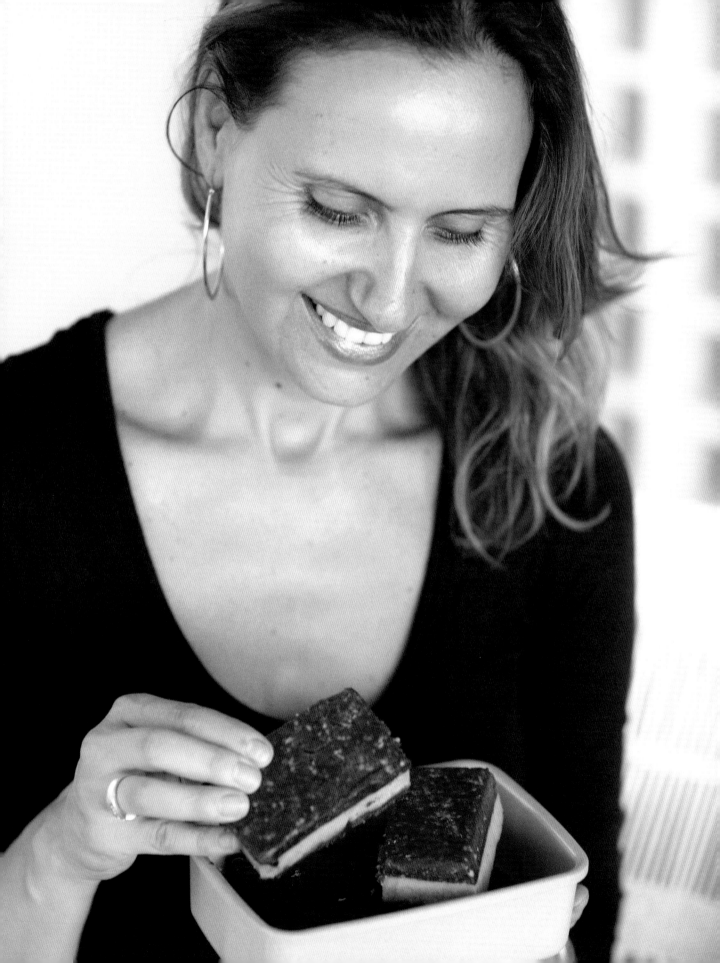

INTRODUCTION

Coconut oil is helping thousands of people all over the world look better, feel better, have more energy and lose weight for good.

A few years ago, I didn't know what coconut oil was. Apart from the occasional junk food 'treat' I considered myself quite healthy. I ate mostly vegetarian food, drank clean water, gave thanks and lived what I thought to be a highly-conscious lifestyle. But I didn't know about real chocolate, green smoothies or raw nutrition. I used olive oil in my cooking without knowing it was unstable and heat sensitive, and put what I thought were 'good' cosmetics and lotions on my skin.

Despite this healthy lifestyle, I didn't feel great. I often felt run down, low in energy and tired. I suffered from serious bouts of eczema on my forearms and feet, and for as long as I could remember I had rashes on my arms and legs from dermatitis. I had a vulnerable immune system and my digestion was weak, with regular bloating and sensitivities, candida and abdominal pain.

My curiosity about raw food nutrition was sparked when I saw David Wolfe, one of the world's leading authorities on nutrition, speak at a health seminar in Fiji back in 2005. It was a massive eye-opener for me. At that time not one raw food restaurant existed in Australia. Today they are popping up everywhere, as are health coaches, nutrition educators and coconut ambassadors.

Introducing coconut oil into my life was a game changer – the missing link. Eating coconut oil daily, using it in all of my cooking and on my skin and practising oil-pulling therapy, became incredibly easy, sustainable and economical. To this day I continue to discover new benefits and new ways of using coconut oil.

Coconut oil became my passion; the more I used it, the healthier I felt and looked. For the first time in years my skin was not covered in bumps, I had energy without experiencing slumps, and I was free from food addictions and cravings. I drank smoothies and ate foods that were full of coconut oil and other good fats. My body started to absorb food nutrients and no longer gave me digestive problems.

For many years we've been conditioned to believe that fat is the enemy – especially coconut oil! Much of the health industry is yet to catch up on the benefits of coconut oil and other good fats known as 'essential fatty acids'. Put simply: those fats and oils that are 'natural', in other words, made in the way that nature intended – are healthy. Those fats that have been hydrogenated, manipulated and synthesised – are toxic.

In this book I explain the difference between oils that are good for you and oils that are not. I recommend completely avoiding the bad ones if you are to get any real, lasting benefits from coconut oil and superfood nutrition.

'Coconut oil became my passion; the more I used it, the healthier I felt and looked. For the first time in years my skin was not covered in bumps, I had energy without experiencing slumps, and I was free from food addictions and cravings. I drank smoothies and ate foods that were full of coconut oil and other good fats. My body started to absorb food nutrients and no longer gave me digestive problems.'

Nature's fats are an essential source of nutrition. This book explains how coconut oil can balance blood sugars, reduce cravings, benefit your skin, your brain, your baby's health, your digestion – and so much more. This book explains the science behind food combining; how to use good fats to help you lose weight; and how to properly absorb nutrients from other natural food sources.

Adding good fats such as coconut oil to your diet is a must for optimum body function. Good fats are a natural source of nourishment, hydration and healing.

This book is about using coconut oil, whole-foods, superfoods and plant-based foods, both raw and cooked, brimming with goodness, to create radiant health. It will show you how to live clean and well with coconut. It's also a recipe book, a compendium of all the ways I obtain my daily dose of coconut oil and live a toxic-free food and beauty regime.

It contains many of my own recipes, as well as contributions from the Coconut Magic team and coconut-conscious friends.

These recipes are simple and healthy, and are designed to help you incorporate more coconut into your daily lifestyle.

Most, but not all recipes, will include coconut oil, or coconut in some way. Some recipes, such as salad dressings, for example, are best made with olive, flax or hempseed oils. I have also included some juice recipes as I believe they are absolutely necessary for good health. I don't juice with coconut oil – I've never tried it and I don't think it will work. (But if you have, please share your experiences with me!)

I am not a nutritional expert – but I did succeed in transforming my own health and lifestyle in a positive way using coconut oil. This book is the result of years spent researching and travelling the world to visit coconut farms and producers, to get the best, most up-to-date information about coconut oil and its uses.

Join me in the journey towards better health, as you switch from toxic oils and lotions to a simple, cost effective, sustainable lifestyle with Coconut Magic.

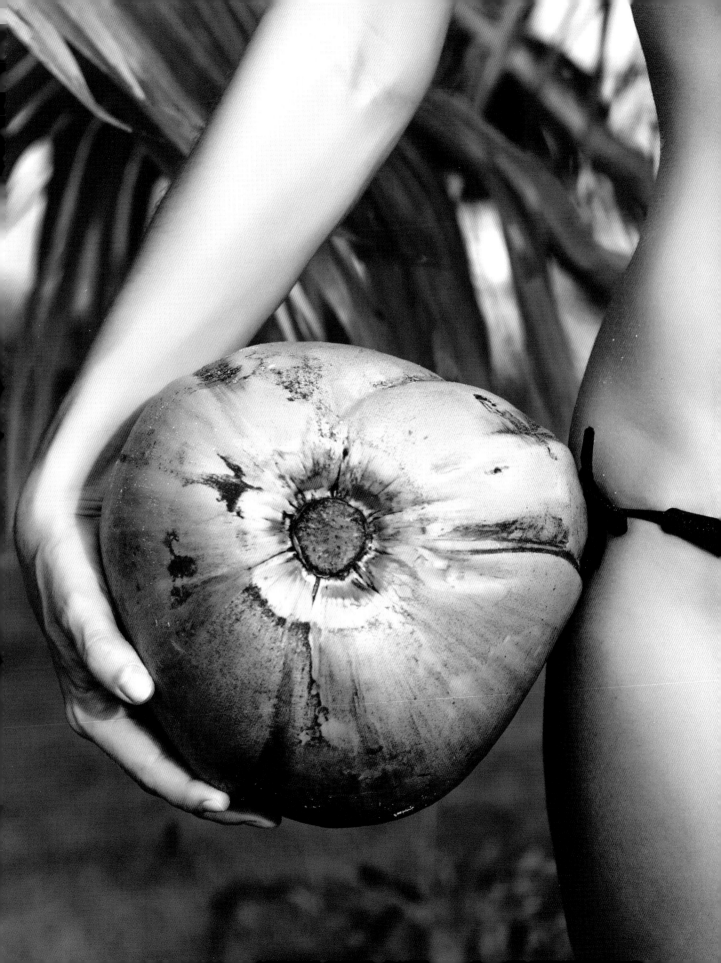

THE HEALTHY COCONUT

_____

The call

The healthy coconut literally called me. I was invited to Thailand by a reputable health retreat with an offer of employment. I felt uncertain about making such a big move, but something inside me said – just go!

I hadn't been there long before I knew something wasn't right. I wasn't happy; I felt trapped and my entrepreneurial spirit was drowning. But I was too afraid to leave. I didn't know what to do – where would I go, how would I earn money? I had just packed up my entire life in Australia, and I couldn't go back. I decided to do what I could to make this job work.

The catalyst

Four weeks later, the Managing Director called me into a meeting. They had made the move for me. 'Pack your things and finish up today,' he said. 'We'll pay you until the end of this week.' I had done nothing wrong – we all knew it was never going to work.

I had made some new friends, so I decided to stay on this beautiful island and try and sort my life out. I felt lost, confused and devastated. Before long the stress started to kick in and my health took a turn for the worst.

My stomach was constantly bloated like a balloon. Even though I was eating little, I had gained a few extra kilos. My skin was breaking out with eczema worse than ever before. Brain fog, headaches, depression and mood swings kicked in. I saw naturopaths, reflexologists and nutritionists.

Strict diets were advised and I struggled with that. Nothing was helping. I went to see a doctor about a serious bout of thrush, which confirmed what the naturopath had said. I had a chronic yeast infection in my digestive tract – candida gone out of control.

Tell me I can't have something and I have to have it – so of course my attempts at dieting were failing. And then one day a local advised me to take some coconut oil. A few days later I received a group email from another friend selling coconut oil. At the foot of the email were some links referencing the health benefits of coconut oil. I started clicking and I started reading – and from that moment, I was hooked. Something so amazing was happening and I knew that life was never going to be the same again.

A few days later I jumped on my scooter to pick up my litre of coconut oil. By this stage I was super excited. I told my friend about my digestive problems, in fact I showed him my bloated stomach and told him about the pain I was experiencing. He gave me my litre of oil and a copy of Dr Bruce Fife's book, *Coconut Cures*. He said: 'Just do what the book says.'

Dr Fife's book talks extensively about the effectiveness of coconut oil in healing many ailments. He recommends a coconut oil detox for chronic digestive issues, in particular yeast, fungal and bacterial infections. His book contains many real-life success stories – some described seeing lumps of candida leaving their body while on the program! The detox is intense – a regimen of between 10 and 15 tablespoons of coconut oil each day, water, and a lemon saltwater mix.

I gave myself two weeks to prepare for the detox, eating mostly raw food and taking the therapeutic dose of three tablespoons per day of coconut oil. As soon as I started to take the coconut oil, its anti-bacterial properties started fighting with my infection and I felt sick. The book described this as a healing crisis, so I expected it – but it was still hard. Thankfully, it lasted only a few days. I applied coconut oil to my skin daily, and three to four times per day to the site of my eczema and dermatitis.

Within two weeks of applying coconut oil to my skin, my rashes, dermatitis and eczema had cleared up. After seven days on the coconut oil detox, taking 10-15 tablespoons of coconut oil per day, I felt that my entire digestion was cleansed and back in balance. I spent the next few weeks slowly introducing all the good foods back into my diet again.

There has not been a day in my life that I have not eaten coconut oil since (even when I attended an ashram in India!). I feel good and I no longer experience the digestive and skin ailments I was once so familiar with.

The mission and the business

I fell in love with coconut oil... coconut everything. I continued to research the benefits, and started to share my experiences. I even phoned my friends and family in Melbourne and told them to start using coconut oil.

Local expats had seen my recovery and were enthused by my passion, which was contagious! They too wanted this 'magic' oil. I started ordering five, 10 and 15 litres at a time for my new 'clients'. I found a mission and a purpose and I loved it. The friend who sold me my first jars declared that something magic had happened...and so my business had a new name: Coconut Magic.

A few weeks later my sister called me from Melbourne. She and her family were not enjoying their coconut oil, and no-one would eat her cooking – the food and the house stank. I couldn't understand how this was happening. She had tried several brands and although they differed, the smell and taste was still just too overpowering to enjoy in their meals.

Together we researched and discovered that each type of coconut oil is made using different processes. My sister came to Thailand and was amazed at the difference in my oil – she could eat this straight from the jar. It was then that I decided it was time to come home to Australia and start importing Coconut Magic.

When I landed back in Australia the only possessions I had were four boxes of books and a couple of bags of clothes – just a few sentimental items that I couldn't bring myself to sell or donate when I'd packed up my life one year earlier. And then there was Mocha, my beautiful six-year-old German Shepherd, who had spent the year with a friend while I was in Thailand. I had missed her so much!

My belongings had been stored in a cupboard in the spare bedroom of my ex-boyfriend's house in West End, Brisbane. Luckily the room was still available and for only $50 per week rent, it became my home for the next 12 months. This, together with the assistance of an investor and the NEISS start-up program, gave me some grounding and potential to focus and start building Coconut Magic.

I had only two litres of coconut oil with me, so I knew I had to get working fast to bring in new business. Not only did I need to fulfill my mission, I also needed an income. Most of all, though, I needed some more of this amazing coconut oil before I ran out!

I didn't start the business with little money. I started the business with no money, no car and just one room to live and work in. I did everything I had to in that one room. I worked countless hours each day and night to fulfill my dream. In a way I think I was so blinded by my own passion and motivation that I kept jumping through the many obstacles that confronted me, ignoring the fears that haunted me.

I knew there was something incredibly special in that 500 ml dark amber glass jar – I knew it each time I looked at it, tasted it and put it on my body.

It took a few months to make a deal with an investor to assist me with the cash to create product labels, a basic website and to make payment for the first import. I still

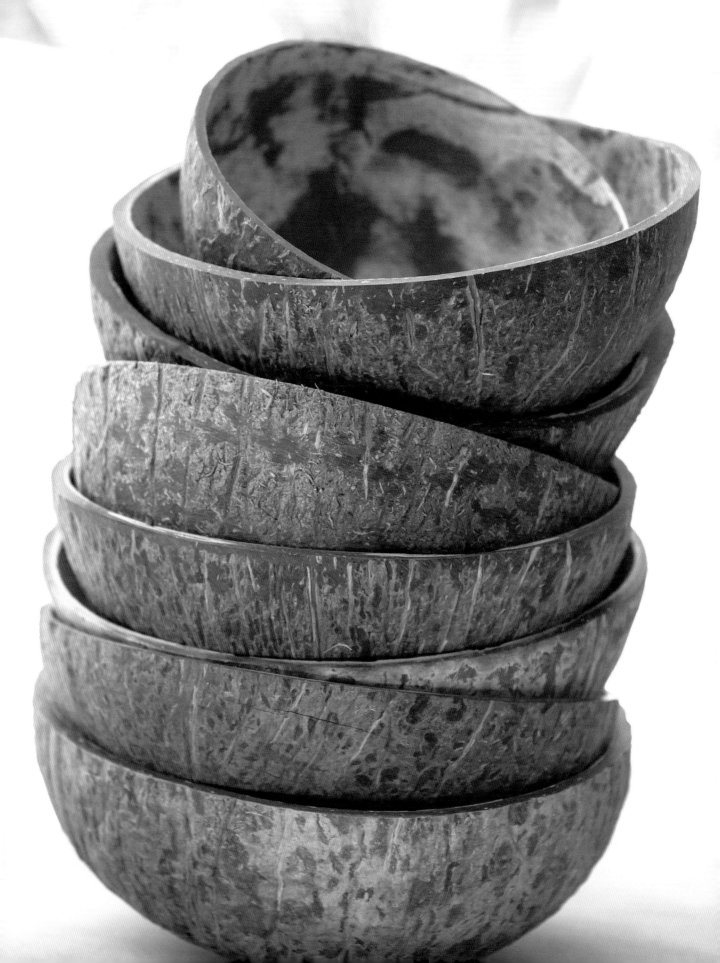

'My goal is to encourage more plant-based food into your chosen diet, to make this transition easy, and to inspire you to look to nature for health, vitality and happiness!'

remember how scared I was when I sent that payment over to Thailand. What if something went wrong, what if they didn't send me the oil, or if it arrived and it was all bad, broken, lost, it didn't get through quarantine? What if I sent the money and never heard from them again? What if no one wanted to buy my coconut oil? I remember many sleepless nights, thinking about the risks I had taken on borrowed money.

I started attending as many networking and health events as possible. Just as my passion spread fast in Thailand, it did also in Australia. People were already anticipating the arrival of this magical coconut oil. I started educating through our Facebook page, and by attending talks. I took every opportunity, whether there were six in the room, or 200. I spoke at raw food community events, eco-friendly community events, small in-house gatherings, health practitioner clinics and networking functions. I shared the amazing benefits of coconut oil and how it had helped me and how it was helping so many others. I explained the difference in quality and the delicate process we use to create our therapeutic, pure-grade coconut oil.

My order arrived and I started to distribute. It was so much fun! I came back to life again just as I had during those initial days of discovery in Thailand. I took stock to my local health stores and offered to do in-store demos. This involved offering people a taste of our coconut oil, and I loved watching their faces light up as they noticed its purity and smooth texture. It was so exciting to see my first jars on the shelves, and even more exciting when the shop manager told me they had sold a few. I could not believe that it was my oil, and people were buying it. My first customer was Go Vita in West End, and then Go Vita in Hawthorne, Brisbane. The word spread and I started doing coconut oil tastings all over Brisbane. It wasn't long before I was ready to order another shipment.

I managed to save up to buy a car – a green, slightly beaten-up Kia Rio 2000 model. I didn't have much choice, but it didn't matter

– it did the job and I was now able to visit more stores and start travelling the coast, both North and South, with Coconut Magic.

In the early days, barely anyone knew about coconut oil, what it was or what it was good for. But in April 2011, a news story on Channel 9's *A Current Affair* dispelled the myth that saturated fat is bad for you. Not only that, the program promoted the benefits of coconut oil! This was just the beginning of a shift in perception about coconut oil and saturated fats in mainstream media. And it's amazing how quickly things have changed since then.

This book explains how you can move from a poor, low-fat diet, filled with cravings and carbohydrates, to a lifestyle rich in healthy fats, with a focus on nutrition, whole foods, raw foods, plant-based foods and, of course, my passion – coconut products.

The glorious yet humble coconut can play a vital role in your transition from processed to whole foods, from disease to well-being.

I will show you how - and why - to incorporate more coconut oil, coconut products, wholefoods and raw foods into your lifestyle, your daily diet, and your skin and hair care regime.

This book will help you replace refined and processed foods, and chemical bathroom products, with cleaner, healthier, toxic-free coconut options.

This book stresses the importance of sourcing the best quality coconut oil and products, and why some fats are better than others. Those who journey with me may find pleasure in continuing to eat animal-based fats, and others the path less travelled and make the move from cow's milk to nut milk, from refined sugar to coconut sweeteners (or honey), and from processed foods to salad and smoothies.

HEALTHY OIL VS TOXIC OIL

The good, the bad and the ugly

If you've been eating the Standard American/Australian Diet (please note the ironic acronym, SAD), then you've probably been consuming low fat, high complex carbohydrate, processed foods. Put simply, this means you've probably been eating a diet consisting of bad fats and too much sugar.

Even if you've been eating well and have avoided the SAD diet, it's important to understand the difference between good fats and bad fats, and the impact of sugar on your metabolism.

The importance of good fats

Fat has had a bad rap for many years; we were told to avoid it because of the risks associated with heart disease and weight gain. Ironically, this low-fat epidemic has seen a massive rise in a multiplicity of diseases of every organ, as well as diabetes, arthritis, gastrointestinal diseases and obesity.

The truth is our body needs good fats to be healthy and thrive – the brain actually needs fat in order to function! The body needs fat to burn fat and good fat is a source of energy.

It is possible to make good fat choices, which can provide us with a wealth of health benefits, essential nutrients, disease prevention and healing, plus the protection of our vital organs. Udo Erasmus wrote an entire book on this: *Fats That Heal, Fats That Kill*. In his book, *Toxic Oils*, David Gillespie conducted some in-depth research on oils and selected Coconut Magic as the best coconut oil available today because of its nutritional profile.

Bad fats, many of which are found in the modern SAD diet, have been linked to cancer, especially cancers of the skin, breast, pancreas and colon. Bad fats cause degenerative diseases, such as heart disease, Alzheimer's and arthritis, as well as lifestyle conditions such as obesity and diabetes. Bad fats are indigestible, leading to excess cholesterol, which is stored in the blood and tissues.

You can see why fat has had such a bad rap!

And yet the path to great health is as simple as replacing trans fats and processed foods with clean fats – fats that are cold pressed, organic and non-hydrogenated.

But before you do, it's vital to understand the difference between good fats and bad fats. Let's start with a quick chemistry lesson.

(Throughout this book I will be referring to both fats and oils. The only difference between the two is that fats are solid and oils are liquid at room temperature. Oils are usually derived from plants, and fats are usually from animals. Both consist of molecules called 'fatty acids'.)

The chemistry of fats

The two main elements of any fats are carbon (C) and hydrogen (H). The basic structure of any fat is a chain of carbon atoms.

In a single bond, carbon has four electrons and must share this with four bonds to be complete.

In a double bond each carbon will contribute at least two electrons with at least one other atom that also contributes two of its electrons.

Fats are classified in two ways: **by saturation and by the length of the fatty acid chain.**

1. Saturation

The molecular structure of the carbon atoms and their bonds categorises fat as either saturated or unsaturated (which can then be further categorised as monounsaturated and polyunsaturated fat).

Saturated fats have no double bonds and are therefore solid at room temperature.

When the bonds are all single, the fat stays very stable and is less prone to oxidation (or breakdown). These are called saturated fats because they contain the maximum number of hydrogens attached to each carbon.

The best saturated fats are derived from plant sources such as coconut oil. Saturated fats can also be derived from animal sources such as grass-fed butter, clarified butter or ghee, pastured lard (pork fat), pastured tallow (beef fat) and duck fat.

Unsaturated fats may have one or more double bond. It's this double bond that causes the chain to bend and consequently become more fragile. The more double bonds a fat contains, the more prone to oxidation it is. These fats are liquid at room temperature.

- A monounsaturated fat has one double bond – for example, olive oil.

- A polyunsaturated fat has more than one double bond – for example vegetable oils, nut oils, seed oils and fish oils.

Polyunsaturated and monounsaturated fats are unstable and are therefore most beneficial when eaten in their cold pressed, organic and raw state. Once these fats are heated, oxidation occurs, the chain is broken down and they can become toxic in the body.

Myths about saturation

Much of the information about saturated fat and cholesterol that has appeared in mainstream media has been inaccurate. In particular, saturated fats have been the target of a host of negative publicity, with claims that eating saturated fat leads to clogging of the arteries. In reality, arterial plaque consists of cooked, unsaturated fats and foreign cholesterol derived from eating animal products.

The health benefits of fats and oils cannot be determined simply by their molecular structure or level of saturation, therefore to claim unsaturated fat as good and saturated fat as bad, is inaccurate.

We have been told that all saturated fat, no matter whether hydrogenated, plant or animal based, was bad. However, it's important to know that the saturated fat in coconut oil is not metabolised in the body in the same way as saturated fats from other sources. So that makes coconut oil and coconut products a good source of saturated fat.

Some unsaturated fats are good for you and some are not. The same goes for saturated fats. (It's more to do with where the oil is extracted from (raw materials), how it is extracted, processed and stored.)

The negative propaganda about coconut oil began in the 1940s when some large multi-national organisations introduced their brand of processed, hydrogenated oils onto the market. Their claims that tropical oils caused heart disease and raised cholesterol created fear; this fear then created a market for their own cheaper cooking oils and fats, such as canola, soya bean and corn oil, as well as margarine.

Sadly their marketing initiatives worked and coconut oil was labelled as an unhealthy saturated fat. And so began the rise in consumption of vegetable oils – and the rise of heart disease, obesity, diabetes, Alzheimer's, arthritis and other forms of degenerative disease. All I can say is, thankfully, we know better now!

In the past four years coconut oil has made a big comeback, as not only the healthiest oil to use for cooking but also as one of the healthiest oils that exists!

Your body needs saturated fat for optimal function. Coconut oil is the healthiest kind of saturated fat that we can consume. Saturated fats are needed for proper function of your cell membranes, liver, immune system, heart, lungs, bones, hormones, satiety (reducing hunger) and genetic regulation.

Coconut oil contains no cholesterol – in fact it may actually help to lower cholesterol levels in the body. In this way it out-performs cold pressed olive oil. People from coconut-eating cultures in the tropics have consistently lower cholesterol levels than people in the West.

Check the ingredients list of packaged foods and avoid all vegetable oils and hydrogenated oil. Look for these names: hydrogenated oil, partially hydrogenated oil, soya bean oil, sunflower, canola oil, trans fat (including less than 1%), vegetable oil, cottonseed oil and palm oil.

Note: Even though palm oil and palmolein have a decent nutritional profile, I personally choose to avoid these for the negative impact their production can have on our wildlife and environment.

Trans fats

Some fats can be artificially manipulated into a saturated state through the man-made process of hydrogenation; these are known as trans fats or trans fatty acids.

Trans fatty acids were created to replace either saturated fats that were in short supply (such as butter during war times) or to replace unstable polyunsaturated fats in processed foods and baked goods, therefore prolonging shelf life.

Basically trans fats were created for the processed food market in order to make more money. And they are incredibly detrimental to your health. (Loopholes in Australian labeling laws have allowed manufacturers to claim a product as 'trans fat free' when in fact the product does contain trans fats. It is therefore best to stick with trusted brands.)

Trans fats increase our risk of heart disease by increasing the 'bad' (LDL) cholesterol, while also lowering the 'good' HDL cholesterol in our blood. LDL cholesterol can build up on the inside of artery walls, contributing to artery blockages that can lead to heart attacks. The higher your LDL cholesterol levels, the higher your risk.

High-density lipoprotein (HDL) cholesterol is known as 'good' cholesterol because it may help prevent arteries from becoming clogged.

Did you know...

Nutritionists commonly refer to fats and oils as 'the good and the bad'. The table on page 19, titled Types of Fats, shows a breakdown of good and bad oils, also listed by their levels of stability. 'Good' but unstable oils can quickly become 'bad' when heated because of their tendency to become rancid. There are only a few oils that are safe enough to use in cooking.

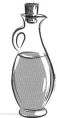

2. Length of fatty acids

As mentioned earlier, fats are classified **by saturation and by the length of the fatty acid chain.**

A fat is categorised as monoglyceride, diglyceride or triglyceride, depending on whether there are one, two, or three fatty acid chains present. The length is determined by the number of carbon atoms they contain, and are classified as short, medium and long chain.

This can be quite complicated, so for our purposes it's enough to know that the length of the chain, the number of double bonds (if any) and their position determine the type of fatty acid present.

For example, lauric acid is the principal fatty acid in coconut oil. None of the bonds between carbon atoms are double, so lauric acid is a natural saturated fat.

Fatty acids with four or six carbons in their chain are known as Short Chain Fatty Acids (SCFAs). Butter is a good example.

Medium chain fatty acids (MCFAs, also known as Medium Chain Triglycerides or MCTs) have eight to 12 carbons in their chains. Most of the fatty acids that make up coconut oil are medium chain.

MCFAs require less energy and fewer enzymes to digest, putting less strain on your digestive system. MCFAs are sent directly to your liver, where they are immediately converted into energy rather than being stored as fat. Therefore, MCFAs actually help stimulate your body's metabolism, aiding to weight loss. For most people, coconut oil can be emulsified during digestion without burdening the liver and the gall bladder. Thus, coconut oil provides more energy more rapidly than most other fat sources.

Fatty acids with 14 or more carbons are called Long Chain Fatty Acids (LCFAs). Most animal fats and vegetable oils are long chain fatty acids. LCFAs are difficult for your body to break down – they require special enzymes for digestion and they put more strain on your pancreas and liver, as well

TYPES OF FATS

Polyunsaturated – unstable	
Not suitable for heating	
The good	The bad
Hempseed oil	Processed vegetable oils such as;
Flax seed oil	Corn oil
Sesame seed oil	Vegetable oils
	Grape seed oil
	Cotton seed oil

Monounsaturated – moderately stable	
Not suitable for heating	
The good	The bad
Avocado oil	Soybean oil
Walnut oil	Peanut oil
Almond oil	Canola oil
Macadamia oil	
Olive oil	

Saturated – stable	
Suitable for heating	
The good	The bad
Coconut oil	Palm oil
Cacao butter	Pasteurised dairy
Butter/Ghee	

NB: To be considered 'good', oils must be organic and cold pressed. Beware of the term 'natural'.

as your entire digestive system. LCFAs are predominantly stored in your body as fat, and can be deposited within your arteries in lipid forms such as cholesterol.

There are a number of good fats we can include in our diet that are extremely beneficial; some are completely essential for good health. Coconut oil remains unique for its incredible health and healing benefits.

The coconut oil difference – the science

It is coconut oil's unique molecular structure that makes it stand apart from all other oils.

Coconut oil contains the following MCFAs (between six and 12 carbon chains):

✔ C12 – Lauric acid

✔ C10 – Capric acid

✔ C8 – Caprylic acid

✔ C6 – Caproic acid

Coconut oil naturally contains all four of the MCFAs and a small percentage of LCFAs.

Lauric acid

About 50% of coconut oil is made up of lauric acid. This is considered to be a 'miracle' ingredient because of its unique health-promoting properties. The body converts lauric acid into monolaurin, which has anti-viral, anti-bacterial and anti-protozoa properties. Monolaurin is a monoglyceride that can actually destroy lipid-coated viruses. Lauric acid has the greatest anti-viral activity and has potent immune enhancing properties.

Lauric acid is only found naturally in mother's breast milk and in coconut oil. This is what gives coconut oil its reputation for being the breast milk of Mother Nature. Lauric acid naturally offers immune building and bacteria protection properties to infants.

Capric acid

Capric acid has strong anti-viral and anti-microbial properties. It is converted into monocaprin in the body, where it can help combat viruses, bacteria and the yeast overgrowth, candida albicans.

Caprylic acid

Caprylic acid is also abundant in coconut oil and is responsible for many of its health benefits, particularly for lactating mothers, and those with diabetes.

MCT oil – fractionated coconut oil

Medium Chain Triglyceride (MCT) oil is a manufactured oil in which the MCFAs are separated from the LCFAs via a process called 'fractionation'. You would think that MCT oil would therefore have more MCFAs – but most MCT oils generally contain only the capra fatty acids; lauric acid is either missing, or present in minuscule amounts. Some people prefer MCT oil because it stays liquid at much lower temperatures – more convenient than coconut oil (you can use it in salad dressings, for example), but it comes without the major benefits of lauric acid, and due to its processing cannot be made organically.

Essential Fatty Acids – EFAs

The body can synthesise most of the fats it needs from your diet. However, two essential fatty acids (EFAs), linolenic and linoleic acid, can only be obtained from food. These basic fats, found in fish, other seafood including algae and krill, and in some plants, nuts and seeds, are used to build specialised fats called omega-3 and omega-6 fatty acids

Coconut oil is made predominantly of MCFA's that provide fuel for the body, it is therefore not classified as an EFA.

Omega-9 (oleic acid) and some other fatty acids are classified as 'conditionally essential', meaning they may be essential in the presence of disease. Omega-9 is essential but technically not an EFA because the human body can manufacture a limited amount, providing that other essential EFAs are present. Monounsaturated oleic acid may help lower heart attack risk and arteriosclerosis, and aid in cancer prevention.

EFAs support the cardiovascular, reproductive, immune and nervous systems. The human body needs EFAs to manufacture and repair cell membranes, enabling the cells to obtain optimum nutrition and expel harmful waste products.

A primary function of EFAs is the production of prostaglandins – a group of lipids that are made at the site of tissue damage or infection. Prostaglandins regulate body functions such as heart rate, blood pressure, blood clotting, fertility and conception, and play a role in immune function by regulating inflammation and encouraging the body to fight infection.

EFAs are also needed for proper growth in children, particularly for neural development and maturation of sensory systems, with male children having higher needs than females. Foetuses and breast-fed infants also require an adequate supply of EFAs through the mother's dietary intake.

Fish oils

Fish oils are a source of polyunsaturated EFAs – however it's important to know the difference between farmed and wild caught fish, if you are eating fish for its health benefits.

Many fish oils nowadays are mass-produced, in whole form and in capsules. Just like coconut oil capsules, you would require ridiculous amounts to get the required intake, and it is virtually impossible to monitor the quality.

Because of the high demand for fish, most of the fish we consume is farmed, and this poses some environmental as well as health concerns. It might surprise you to know that there are many breeds of fish that contain higher levels of toxins than red meat. This is because many thousands of fish are tightly packed together in tanks or cages. They are fed fish food or fish-meal tablets, rather than food from natural sources. These conditions breed disease and parasites such as sea lice, which requires the fish and their

> **'Coconuts are one of the greatest gifts on this planet. No matter where you are, what you have done, how much you have mistreated your body, fresh coconut and coconut oil can improve your health and well-being.'**

environment to be treated with antibiotics and fungicides.

Salmon cage farms drop as much sewage into the sea as a city of 1,000 people. With as much as 50,000 fish in a two-acre space, that's a lot of fish poop! Therefore farmed fish and fish oils are not considered clean oils.

Research shows that farmed fish has less usable omega-3 fatty acids than wild-caught fish and a 20% lower protein content. Farmed fish are fattier and have a high concentration of omega-6 fatty acids. It's important to know that an imbalance in the levels of omega-3 and omega-6 fatty acids creates inflammation in the body.

Some salmon farmers add synthetic pigments to create a nice pink salmon – wild salmon get their colour naturally by feeding on krill.

Oil for vitality – good, clean fats are vital

Good fats are vital in our diets, and that's why I recommend using coconut oil every day.

Coconut oil offers natural anti-bacterial, anti-fungal, anti-viral and anti-microbial benefits, but there are some other sources of good oils and fats as well, including: flaxseeds, flaxseed meal, evening primrose seeds, hempseed oil, hempseeds, walnuts, pumpkin seeds, Brazil nuts, sesame seeds, avocados, some dark leafy green vegetables (kale, spinach, purslane, mustard greens, collards, etc), and wheat germ oil. These all provide good plant-based sources of pure EFAs.

Oil from flax and chia seeds provide the highest linolenic (omega-3) content of any seed. One tablespoon per day of flaxseed oil provides the recommended daily adult dose of omega-3 (depending on individual body weight).

Some of the recipes in this book include flax oil, hemp-seed oil, hempseeds, raw nuts, extra virgin olive oil, cacao butter, acai berry powder and chia seeds, as these all offer a great combination and balance of omega-3, omega-6 and omega-9 EFAs. They are also delicious and easy to include in a raw food dessert, salad or smoothie.

In today's western SAD diet, we suffer from an imbalance of EFAs – we are eating too much omega-6 and not enough omega-3 and saturated fat. What's worse, we're eating rancid, oxidized omega-6 oils such as safflower, canola, vegetable, soybean and peanut oil – all the common cooking oils – which have been linked to many cardiovascular and degenerative diseases today.

Coconut oil helps to increase the uptake of EFAs and fat soluble vitamins in the body's cells. When you eat coconut oil together with the omega oils from EFAs, you increase your body's absorption of the omegas by 100%. So it makes sense to eat your good fats all together either in a meal or a smoothie – you'll get much better absorption of vital nutrients.

Keeping a good, clean fat balance may look something like this:

✓ Ingest coconut oil as a daily dose for its therapeutic healing benefits.

✓ Use coconut oil in all cooked dishes for its stability, and pour hemp, olive and/or flaxseed oil over a cold dish or salad.

✓ Use nuts and seeds in raw desserts, bliss balls, nut milks, or simply enjoy them on their own as a snack.

✓ Eat Coconut Magic raw energy bars! They are made with nuts, seeds and coconut oil – a great combination of healthy oils with raw superfood flavours such as coconut, cacao, raspberry and chai spice.

Go for the glow!

Excellent sources of omega-3 include chia, flax and hempseeds. Flax and chia seeds are best consumed when freshly ground.

Virgin coconut oil, and the entire coconut is known as a catalyst for omega-3 absorption. So it is a great idea to combine these nutritious raw fat sources in food recipes, and go for the glow!

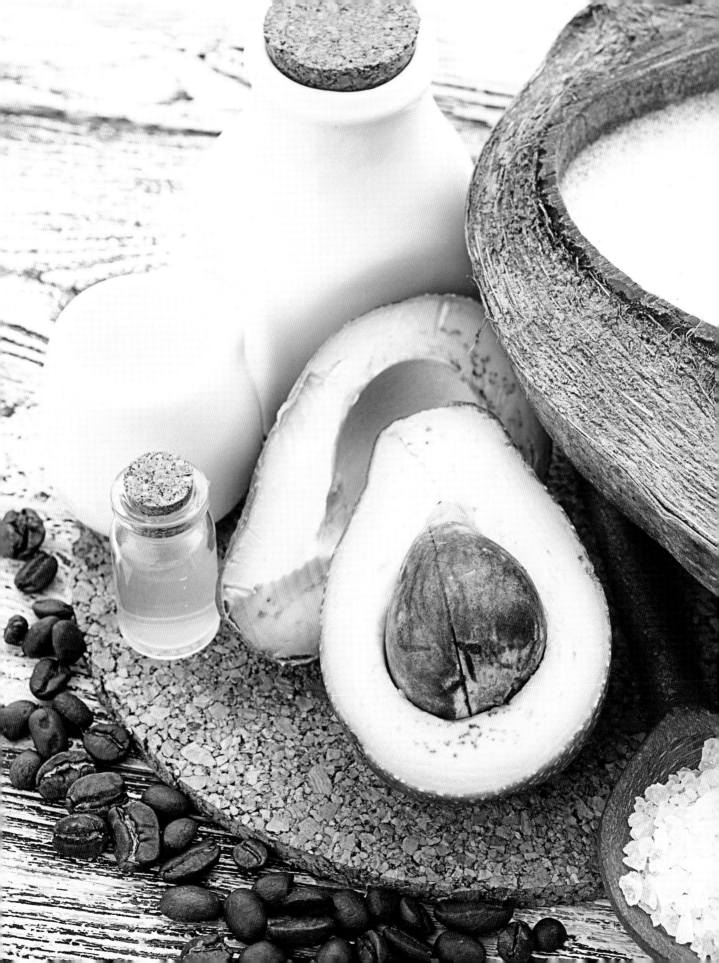

NATURAL SUGAR VS PROCESSED SUGARS

As previously mentioned, the SAD diet consists of an overload of bad fats and sugar. So what's the problem with sugar? David Gillespie summarised this in his book, *Sweet Poison:* Sugar is highly addictive and toxic.

Sugar disables your immune system, promoting fat storage and weight gain. It is known to promote insulin resistance and a host of other health-related issues. Researchers claim it is more addictive than cocaine, which is why food manufacturers like to have lots of it in their processed foods – not just because it's cheap, but also because it keeps you addicted to their products.

In summary, sugar suppresses your immune system, is fattening, ageing and addictive.

Sweeteners such as refined sugar and high fructose corn syrup don't contain any vital nutrients and therefore supply 'empty' calories.

What's the difference between sucrose, glucose and fructose?

Sucrose, the technical name for table sugar, cane sugar or white sugar, is made of one glucose molecule and one fructose molecule bound together. Fructose is a simple sugar that occurs naturally in foods. It can only be metabolised by the liver and can't be used for energy by your body, whereas glucose (also known as dextrose) is absorbed directly into the bloodstream during digestion and acts as an instant source of energy.

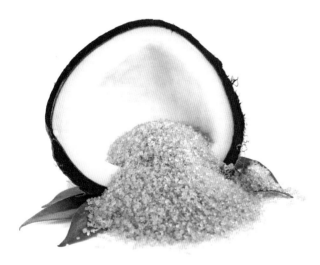

There are now many natural sweeteners available that can offer you nutritional value and a sweet kick that won't spike your blood sugar levels. These include:

Coconut flower nectar

Coconut flower nectar is one of the lowest glycemic index sweeteners on the market. It comes from the sap collected from the flower blossom of the coconut palm tree. When the flower is sliced, the nectar is captured, watered down and gently boiled. It forms a syrup-like consistency as the nectar crystallises. The process is minimal and nothing artificial is added.

At the time of collection the fructose level of the nectar

is approximately 1.5%. By the end of the process it is around 10%. This is still much lower than the 80 or 90% levels of fructose in most other sweeteners.

Coconut sugar

The nutritional profile of coconut sugar and coconut nectar are the same. The consistency and the taste however are different.

Coconut sugar and coconut nectar both have an extremely low glycemic index (GI) of 35. A low GI is important for everyone, especially diabetics, those experiencing energy slumps, or wishing to lose weight.

The nutrient-rich coconut sap from the coconut palm is naturally abundant in:

- ✓ 17 amino acids, the building blocks of protein

- ✓ Broad-spectrum B vitamins, especially Inositol, known for its effectiveness in treating depression, high cholesterol, inflammation and diabetes

- ✓ Vitamin C

- ✓ Minerals, particularly potassium, essential for electrolyte balance, the regulation of high blood pressure and sugar metabolism

- ✓ FOS (fructo-oligosaccharide) – a prebiotic that assists digestive health.

The United Nations 'Food and Agriculture Organization' (FAO) has reported that coconut palm sweeteners are the single most sustainable sweetener in the world. Coconut palms grow in diverse, wildlife-supportive agro-ecosystems. They can help restore damaged soils, and require little water for production. Coconut palms produce an average of 50-75% more sugar per acre than sugar cane.

Coconut sugar has long been a staple of South East Asian cuisine and herbal medicine. It has yet to be commercialised, so it is still farmed predominantly by small farm holdings rather than giant corporations.

The sap of the coconut tree produces a multitude of delicious products, including our own brand of Coconut Cider Vinegar, Coconut Aminos Seasoning Sauce, Coconut Nectar, and Coconut Crystals, all of which are made following raw food principles by either ageing the sap for up to a year, or evaporating it at low temperatures after it is collected. However, neither coconut nectar nor coconut sugar is technically considered to be 'raw'. Both have become favourite sweeteners within raw food communities due to their taste, low GI levels and impressive nutritional profiles compared with honey and agave.

I have personally visited the farmers that produce our coconut sugar and coconut nectar. It is a beautiful process to watch as generations of family members follow suit in the farming and production of this natural and organic coconut product.

'I see a lot of 'health products' sweetened with raw, organic cane sugar. Do not let the fancy words deceive you – this is just sugar. Your liver does not know the difference between cane, brown, raw or organic. It is still simply a sugar.'

LOW-DOWN ON SUGARS

Good coconut sweeteners:

Coconut Sugar and Coconut Nectar

- Is a natural product
- Rich in minerals, particularly iron, zinc, calcium and potassium
- Contains short chain fatty acids, polyphenols and antioxidants that may also provide some health benefits
- Low GI of 35
- Can contain between 70-80% sucrose
- Contains a fibre known as Inulin, which may slow glucose absorption.

Better-than-sugar sweeteners:

Honey

- Is a natural product
- Contains beneficial anti-bacterial properties
- Contains about 17% water (water has no calories)
- Consists of about 1.5g of sucrose; the rest is fructose and glucose. Glucose is absorbed quickly, giving the body an immediate boost of energy, while fructose has a slower rate of absorption. Therefore honey offers both an immediate and sustained energy boost particularly if you're participating in sports
- Contains some vitamins (particularly Vitamin C, Niacin, Folate, Pantothenic Acid, Choline and Betain)
- Contains quality proteins
- Contains small amounts of minerals (sugar has none)
- GI of 55.

Maple Syrup

- Is a natural product
- Has less fructose than honey, but is still 60-70% sucrose
- Contains minerals including iron, calcium, zinc, manganese, potassium and sodium
- Contains around 24 antioxidants; the darker the maple syrup, the more antioxidants it contains.
- GI of 54.

Stevia

- Is a natural product
- Contains no calories
- Does not cause cavities
- Stevia in its unprocessed form may contain proteins, fibers, carbohydrates, iron, phosphorus, calcium, potassium, sodium, magnesium, zinc and vitamins A and C. In its processed, powder or liquid form, it probably has none of these.
- Stevia may cause adverse reactions in some people, including dizziness, bloating, muscle pain and numbness, and may act as a diuretic.

CHOOSING YOUR COCONUT OIL

Which coconut oil is best?

There are many types of coconut oil on the market today: virgin, extra virgin, expeller pressed, refined, unrefined, organic, and even a 'tasteless' variety.

I am often asked to explain the difference between virgin coconut oil and extra virgin coconut oil. The answer is simple: there is no difference. Coconut oil is either virgin or non-virgin.

There are no commonly understood or accepted definitions for 'extra' virgin coconut oil, as there are, for example, in the olive oil industry. A coconut oil producer may refine their oil, or include an additional process to alter the taste – they may then label this oil as 'extra' virgin coconut oil.

Having visited many different coconut farms and tasted coconut oil samples from all over the world, I have found that the gentle and unique extraction process we use to make Coconut Magic virgin coconut oil is by far the most superior in taste, texture and aroma. It tastes and smells beautiful, and leaves no offensive after-taste. It absorbs easily into your skin, and is delicious in all cooked and raw food recipes.

Therapeutic-grade oils

I first met Barbara at a presentation I did in Brisbane in 2012. Barbara had many dental problems, including four root canals and two crowns. She had pain and inflammation from an ongoing, low-grade infection in her mouth. Part of my presentation was on oil pulling therapy (see page 58 for more information). Barbara bought some Coconut Magic coconut oil for her dental health.

A few years later Barbara called our office about an online order she had placed. She told me that after our initial meeting, and only one week after beginning the practice of oil pulling, she experienced great relief and healing in her mouth. She continues to oil pull using Coconut Magic, and has no dental health problems or inflammation in her gums.

This underlined to me the difference between oil, and therapeutic-grade oil.

Lauric acid content

Contrary to popular belief, the lauric acid content of a coconut does not determine its quality. Organic virgin coconut oil is the coconut oil at its most natural state, so the content of lauric acid in each coconut will vary from day to day and reflect the content of its unique raw materials, the coconut meat.

The benefits of coconut oil come from its medium chain fatty acid profile (of which lauric acid is a part), and the fact that coconut oil is over 93% saturated fat. This means that, unlike other oils, coconut oil does not oxidise and retains 93% of its antioxidant properties.

Taste the difference

The taste of coconut oil will differ with each brand for a number of reasons: the quality of the soil, the types of coconuts used, where the coconuts come from, the process of extraction and the packaging.

The traditional quick dry, expeller-pressed or fermentation methods mostly used across the Pacific Islands and the Philippines will generally have a stronger flavour. This is because of the heat used to dry out the moisture from the coconut meat.

The coconut oil production process

When I returned home to Australia after my one-year adventure in Thailand, I wanted to share and spread the magic of coconut oil with the world and I wanted to make it a commercially viable business.

So to learn more about what was available for purchase, I sourced coconut oil samples from every part of the world – from Indonesia, Sri Lanka, Vanuatu, Fiji, Solomon Islands, Philippines and India. I even sampled other brands of oil from Thailand.

They were all very different. They differed dramatically in taste, colour, smell, texture and price. I tried them all, but I simply couldn't enjoy them the way I enjoyed Coconut Magic, which stood out from the crowd in terms of smell, taste, clarity and texture. So it was an easy decision to stay with my original choice.

I also investigated our manufacturing process to learn all I could about this amazing oil. Our process was developed by the founding family together with a food scientist, in order to produce a premium quality coconut oil that maintains its purity and therapeutic properties during processing.

Our process is completely sustainable, and uses no chemicals, no hexane, no direct heat and no dehydration – just a very gentle, cold pressed, separation technique.

Coconut Magic – the premium quality difference

There are a number of reasons why Coconut Magic coconut oil holds the premium brand status – and it all starts at production.

Raw materials

Our coconuts are grown in quality-controlled, certified organic coconut farms in Thailand. The total plantation area stretches across 450 hectares in a collection amongst a range of gorgeous Thai provinces. The farms are all maintained with sustainability in mind, using decomposable glass and natural fertilisers such as fallen coconut leaves and cow dung. Thai soil is also known for its high mineral content.

Our coconuts grow on flat farming land and can therefore be harvested regularly. This is not the case in many island nations, where coconut farmers tend to harvest all the coconuts (regardless of their state of maturity) in one specific harvesting period, due to difficulties in transportation on tougher terrain.

Production process

Once the coconuts are shelled and the coconut meat is washed, we run a stringent quality control process whereby inferior raw materials are discarded and sent off to produce low-grade or refined coconut oils for other markets. We eliminate coconuts that are mouldy or smell bad, rejecting damaged, cracked or old coconuts, or coconuts that have started to ferment or sprout.

To process Coconut Magic oil, we use a unique, ultra-cold centrifuge extraction method that involves extracting the oil at freezing temperatures to lock in the freshness and maintain the essence of the fresh coconuts. No direct heat and no chemicals are used. (Some processes remove all of the coconut flavour, leaving the oil odourless and bland. I refer to this as oil that has had the 'guts' removed. Although soft and mild, our coconut oil maintains its integrity.)

Speed is of the essence in the next part. We select the purest raw materials, then pour into dark amber glass jars (or BPA-free plastic for bulk containers). This takes just a few hours, within controlled conditions, which minimizes the risk of bacteria and foreign objects getting into the oil. This way we eliminate the production of mould or premature rancidity.

Our oil is exported already sealed and packaged, so we can maintain quality control measures during transit.

To produce one 500 ml jar of Coconut Magic pure coconut oil, we have cold pressed seven to eight mature coconuts.

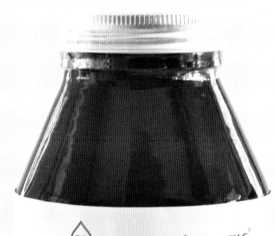

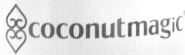

coconutmagic

Raw Organic
Virgin Coconut Oil
Cold Pressed & Pure

energy • health • beauty

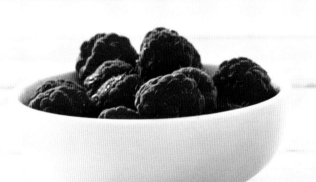

which coconut oil do I choose?

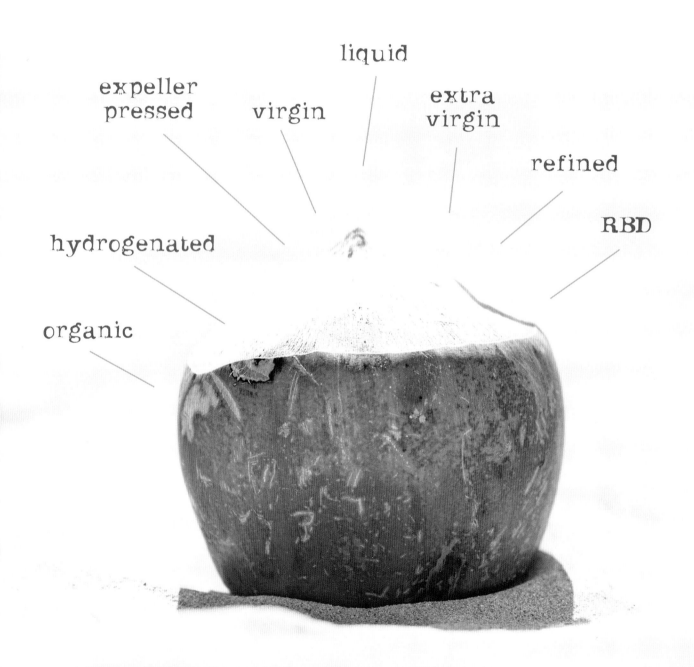

expeller pressed

virgin

liquid

extra virgin

refined

RBD

hydrogenated

organic

TIPS ON CHOOSING YOUR COCONUT OIL

Before you can choose the oil that's right for you, you need to understand how coconut oil is made.

There are different ways of extracting coconut oil from the meat or kernel of the coconut. Pressing the coconut is one of the simplest and most efficient ways of extracting oil.

1. Non-Virgin Coconut Oil

RBD (Refined, Bleached and Deodorised): Coconuts are dried in the sun, sometimes for weeks at a time (or in a faster process, by direct heat) to make copra, which at this stage is inedible, as it contains dust particles, insect remains, microbes, fungal spores and many other substances that may be harmful for health.

The copra is then heated to very high temperatures and pressed to produce crude coconut oil. Then sodium hydroxide is added to it and it is further filtered using clay or diatomaceous earth to remove the mono-fats or free fats. The oil is then deodorised using steam and a vacuum process.

If clay is used in the filtering process, the oil can be certified organic.

Crude coconut oil made from copra and RBD: Coconuts that are mouldy or damaged, or that have started to ferment or sprout are processed into crude oil, which is then pressed and filtered, then refined, bleached and deodorised. It its crude state, it smells and tastes really bad, which is why it needs to be refined.

These lower quality raw materials can also be fractionated to make MCT oil or liquid coconut oil. Both are made from copra.

Producers use this method because it is cheaper and higher yields can be produced. The quality is inferior to a virgin coconut oil which only uses premium raw coconut materials.

MCT oil or fractionated coconut oil liquid: The lauric acid content is removed, leaving the capric and caprylic acid content. MCT oil has some health benefits, even though the most beneficial MCFA, lauric acid, has been removed.

MCT oil is never organic because no organic certifying body will accept it as an organic product. It has something to do with the process, and the fact that the copra materials being used are not organic.

Hydrogenated: This is a process that produces trans fatty acids. This creates a long shelf life and ironically, a product that feels good in your mouth. Most coconut oil producers do not use this method.

Beware of cheap blends labelled 'virgin' or 'organic'. In order to keep up with the demand of a growing market, some producers may blend their cold pressed oil with 50% RBD oil. This allows them to produce much higher yields and also cut production costs in half.

Unfortunately labeling laws do not regulate this type of blend and manufacturers can still call this virgin, unrefined and raw cold pressed – and even organic. It is therefore important for you to know how to find high quality oil.

2. Virgin Coconut Oil (VCO)

Within the APPC (Asian Pacific Coconut Community) the definition of virgin is fairly general:

'Virgin coconut oil (VCO) is obtained from fresh and mature kernel (12 months old from pollination) of the coconut

(Cocos nucifera L.) by mechanical or natural means with or without the application of heat, which does not lead to alteration of the nature of the oil.

'VCO has not undergone chemical refining, bleaching or deodorising. It can be consumed in its natural state without the need for further processing.

'Virgin coconut oil consists mainly of medium chain tryglycerides, which are resistant to peroxidation. The fatty acids in virgin coconut oil are distinct from animal fats which contain mainly long chain saturated fatty acids.

'Virgin coconut oil is colorless, free of sediment with a natural fresh coconut scent. It is free from rancid odour or taste.'

VCO is produced from the first pressing of the coconut meat. No chemicals are added to refine the coconut oil or to modify its taste. As a result, all of the nutrients remain intact. However, heat may still be used during the process of extraction, and this means the coconut oil will lose some of its specific taste and flavor. If the oil has been subjected to high heat it may have a stronger, more pungent smell and taste, and/or a yellow colour.

Quick dry method: This is the most common way to mass-produce inexpensive coconut oil. The fresh coconut meat is quick-dried using high heat, and then the oil is pressed out via mechanical means.

Centrifuge extraction: The coconut milk is finely spun so that the oil separates, in much the same way that cream separates from dairy milk. The oil then passes through a series of centrifuges until pure oil is obtained. The temperature never rises above 41˚C.

Centrifuge-extracted oil has a mild aroma and delicate taste, due to the absence of high heat in the extraction process.

a. Centrifuge – wet-milling: The oil is extracted from fresh coconut meat without drying first. No direct heat is applied at all. Coconut milk is expressed first by pressing.

The oil is then gently separated from the water. This is the process we have developed and use.

What is left is a pure-grade oil with the full integrity of the coconut essence.

b. Centrifuge – vacuum evaporation: When the moisture is sucked out of the coconut oil, the aroma of coconut also evaporates. Just as with essential oils, the aroma of the coconut oil is actually the essential oil of the coconut, a type of very short chain fatty acid, which can vaporise easily.

What is left is the remaining fatty acids with no coconut aroma, and this makes it a less 'natural' oil.

Direct Micro Expelling (DME): This is a process in which the oil is pressed mechanically. Because no heat is applied, it can be referred to as cold pressed, however there is always friction caused by the movement of the press, which can cause high amounts of heat to be emitted.

De-husked, fully-mature coconuts are split in half and the flesh is grated and dried on the stainless steel surface of a 'flat-top' drier, fuelled with coconut shell. The coconut is dried for about half an hour and then the oil is pressed out via a manually-operated press.

The whole process takes less than an hour and this virgin coconut oil retains good flavour and aroma. This oil is very stable and has a long shelf life.

Fermentation: The fermentation method is used in the Philippines and other parts of Asia. The coconut milk is heated for 36-48 hours then left overnight to allow the heavier liquid to fall to the bottom; the lighter liquid floats to the top. Small curds form in the oil and these are separated by the application of more heat. The oil must be stirred during this process so that the temperature doesn't reach boiling point. The oil is then carefully scooped off to be filtered and bottled.

Fermenting is considered to be the 'poor man's coconut oil' – it's how traditional, home-made coconut oil was made. It's quite labour-intensive and tends to have a limited shelf life, however it is a cheaper method of production.

Look for these things in your coconut oil:

✓ High quality coconut oil should be snow-white in colour when solid, and crystal-clear when liquid

✓ Yellow or grey nuances are signs of inferior quality

✓ You should be able to smell the scent of coconut. The lack of scent means that the oil has been highly processed, has been chemically treated or is refined

✓ Good quality coconut oil is light rather than dense and heavy

✓ When cooked, good coconut oil should be mild and have no strong flavour to it.

The best way to select a good-quality coconut oil is to sample it yourself. Just like a good-quality olive oil, the taste and the smell will reflect its purity and quality.

If it stinks or it makes you gag, don't use, and don't buy it!

I met Sally at an in-store demonstration I was doing. She told me she was taking a spoonful of coconut oil every morning, even though it was making her gag – she was forcing herself to do it, because she knew it was good for her.

I told her that she didn't have to suffer, gave her a sample of Coconut Magic – and watched her eyes light up! She loved it!

A good-quality 'clean' coconut oil, will not taste or smell offensive or over-powering. It will be mild and smooth with a natural, subtle hint of coconut aroma and flavour.

Coconut oil is made up of mostly medium chain fatty acids (MCFAs), which are readily absorbed by the skin. So as well as tasting, test it on your skin! Coconut oil that doesn't absorb easily can be a sign of an inferior or blended oil, because the MCFA content is reduced. Coconut oil that absorbs well is a good sign of a big concentration of MCFAs, which contain most of the coconut's health and healing properties.

In summary, the highest quality oils are determined by:

The raw materials: While coconut water is best made with the young coconut, coconut oil is best made from the mature coconut. This is because the mature coconut – one that is harvested after 12 months – allows for the full maturation of the MCFAs. It is these fatty acids that hold the health properties of coconut oil.

The extraction method: Cold pressed, unrefined, gently extracted without the use of any direct heat will ensure that the oil maintains its full nutritional composition.

Packaging and transportation:

It is also important to consider how the oil is transported after production. The best way to protect coconut oil is to transport it in dark glass. This will ensure that the oil is safe from major temperature fluctuations, undergoes minimal handling and is sealed off from exposure to toxins.

Larger production facilities will import their oil inside containers, and transit time can often be up to six weeks. There is little or no temperature control at this time, and as the oil is moved from its tropical country of origin to its final destination, there is no quality control or protection. Once the oil arrives to its final destination, it is melted and packaged into its various-sized jars or containers. This can create additional exposure to bacteria and other potentially harmful substances while the oil is in transit and being decanted.

You get a better result when the oil is packaged prior to transport; this ensures minimal handling and better temperature control.

NUTRITIVE BENEFITS OF VIRGIN COCONUT OIL

How much coconut oil should I eat?

Doctors and health professionals generally recommend three to five tablespoons per day for optimal benefits. In my experience it depends on what you're trying to achieve. For hormone or blood sugar balance, one tablespoon in the morning and one in the afternoon helps. For weight loss, one tablespoon taken at the beginning of each meal will help burn up the kilojoules of that meal for up to 48 hours. To curb sugar cravings, eat one tablespoon each time you feel that sugar-fix buzz kick in, and the craving should disappear.

Coconut oil is considered medicinal, and experts such as Dr Bruce Fife recommend therapeutic doses to treat specific ailments such as Irritable Bowel Syndrome (IBS), yeast infection, Alzheimer's, diabetes and kidney stones, where much higher doses, up to 10-15 tablespoons per day may be required.

Children will benefit from one to two teaspoons in the morning.

Can I eat too much coconut oil?

If you're new to coconut oil, it's a good idea to start with one tablespoon in the morning and gradually build up to three or five over a few weeks. Your body will tell you when it has had too much coconut oil – you may feel nauseous or have loose stools. Because of the strong cleansing effects, natural anti-bacterial, anti-fungal and anti-viral properties of coconut oil, your body may experience a healing crisis when you first start to consume coconut oil. This is an important part of the detox process, as your body starts to heal by ridding itself of toxins. At this time, reduce the amount you are eating until your body readjusts – this may only take a few days. See it through and you can then build up to the recommended daily therapeutic dose of three to five tablespoons per day, and enjoy!

Simple ways to take your daily dose of coconut oil:

✓ Eat it straight from the jar

✓ Replace your regular cooking oils with coconut oil

✓ Add a tablespoon in your herbal and green teas

✓ Add a tablespoon in your coffee

✓ Add it to your smoothies

✓ Use it on your body for skin hydration and moisture

✓ Coconut oil can replace or compliment any bathroom, skin or beauty care regime.

> ### Take note
>
> Health professionals and advocates of coconut oil recommend three to five tablespoons per day as your daily therapeutic dose.

HOW TO USE COCONUT OIL

Health & Well-Being

Stress relief
Fitness
Digestion
Nose bleeds
Weight loss
Control cravings
Balance blood sugar
Breast-feeding
Energy boost
Mental clarity
Boost metabolism
Cold-sore treatment
Soothe burns
Improve digestion
Thyroid support
Fight yeast, fungus and candida
Balance hormones
Brain health
Oral health
Swimmers' ear

Body & Beauty

Personal hygiene
Body wash, bath oil
Deodorant
Mouthwash
Eye cream
Nail cream
Body moisturiser
Hair conditioning treatment
Eye make-up remover
Lip balm
Massage oil
Heal cuts and skin problems
Eczema
Personal lubricant
Stretch mark prevention
Body scrub

More details about the specific uses for coconut oil, and detailed health-related treatments with coconut oil can also be found on our website: www.coconutmagic.com

Coconut oil capsules

Some people don't like the taste of coconut oil and prefer to take capsules instead. Things to be aware of here include:

1. Dosage: The recommended dose for coconut oil is one tablespoon, three times per day, sometimes even more. One tablespoon is equal to 15 ml of coconut oil, and 15 ml of coconut oil weighs 14 grams.

There are two common sizes of soft gel capsules – 500 mg and 1,000 mg. In order to consume one tablespoon of coconut oil, which is 14 grams, you will need to take 14 x 1,000 mg or 28 x 500 mg soft gel capsules!

2. Quality: You cannot determine the quality of the oil from the label. The manufacturer can put any grade of coconut oil in the capsule and sell it as 'cold pressed raw organic virgin coconut oil'. You could, of course, open up a capsule and conduct a taste test!

Real food is not supposed to be processed or packaged into capsules! That's not conducive to a natural, healthy lifestyle. Let's keep food whole and as close to the way nature intended it to be. If you are having a problem with the taste of coconut oil we don't recommend you buy coconut oil capsules. Instead, we recommend Coconut Magic for its light delicious taste and texture.

Are there adverse side-effects from consuming coconut oil?

Coconut oil has no known side effects. However, if you are used to a low-fat diet, a common adverse reaction could be diarrhea, so it's probably advisable to start with a small amount in the beginning. Why not spread the recommended amount over the course of one day, building up to a larger dose on subsequent days, when your body has adjusted.

DIET & LIFESTYLE CHOICES

Coconut oil is a vital part of many healthy lifestyles:

Vegan, vegetarian

These diets use plant-based foods, such as vegetables, fruits, legumes, nuts, seeds and whole grains. A vegan diet includes no animal products. Most vegetarian diets will include dairy and eggs.

Juices and smoothies

You can add coconut oil, water, cream or milk to your smoothies.

I am often asked: 'Is it better to drink juices or smoothies?' I think it's best to drink both rather than either/or, because both have unique and enormous health benefits.

Smoothies are a combination of whole foods blended together into a drink. Unlike juicing, the foods retain their fibre as well as their vital nutrients. Blending raw fruits and vegetables breaks them down into particles that are easily assimilated by the body. This is especially important, considering the fact that many of us do not chew well enough and/or have compromised digestion.

Blending foods also allows you to introduce new foods and superfoods into your diet, and it's a great way to consume higher amounts of whole foods and superfoods in one simple drink.

A fresh juice is like ingesting a massive amount of life-force and nutrition into your body in one big gulp. It's best to drink fresh juice on an empty stomach. The intense source of nutrition from the fruits and vegetables juiced will enter your blood stream within about 20 minutes.

The Paleo diet

The Paleo diet is a lifestyle where processed foods are avoided. The name comes from the word Paleolithic, which refers to the cave man who didn't have a local supermarket to buy his food from. Instead, he hunted and ate what was in season and what was easily digestible, without processing. Therefore legumes, dairy, vegetable oils and grains are all avoided; instead, meat, saturated fats (from animals and plants) non-starchy vegetables, nuts, eggs and a little low-sugar fruit are preferred.

Paleo advocates love everything about the coconut and include coconut milk, oil, flour, nectar, flakes and chips, in many of their recipes.

Raw food

The raw food diet is based on the belief that the most health-giving food for the body is uncooked. Although most food is eaten raw, heating food is acceptable as long as the temperature stays below 41 degrees Celsius, although this cut-off temperature varies amongst the different raw food communities.

Enzymes are the life force of a food, and they help us digest that food and absorb its nutrients. Raw foodists believe that enzymes are destroyed during cooking or processing, and the body has to compensate by manufacturing its own. Over time, this is thought to lead to digestive problems, nutrient deficiency, accelerated ageing and weight gain.

I highly support eating a diet high in raw foods to maintain nutrition and proper digestion. Raw salads, smoothies, juices and desserts help bump up the ratio of raw versus cooked food on a daily basis.

The raw food diet includes an abundance of coconut oil, coconut meat, dried coconut and coconut nectar in both savory and sweet dishes. Although coconut nectar is not technically raw it is a popular natural sweetener within raw food communities because

of its minimal processing, low Glycemic Index and impressive nutritional profile compared to other natural sweeteners.

Superfoods

What makes a superfood 'super' is the fact that it is filled with nutrition and will help you to feel super healthy. Superfoods are nutrient powerhouse functional foods. They contain particularly large doses of antioxidants, polyphenols, vitamins and minerals, that when consumed regularly have tremendous health benefits.

Superfoods include blueberries, goji berries, hempseed, cacao beans (raw chocolate), maca, spirulina, bee products, and a host of others.

Whole foods

Whole foods are foods that are as close to their natural form as possible; they are processed and refined as little as possible before being consumed.

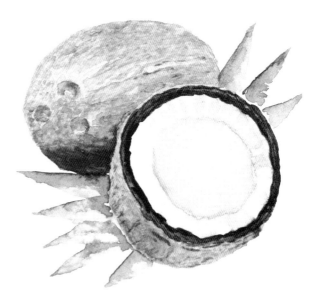

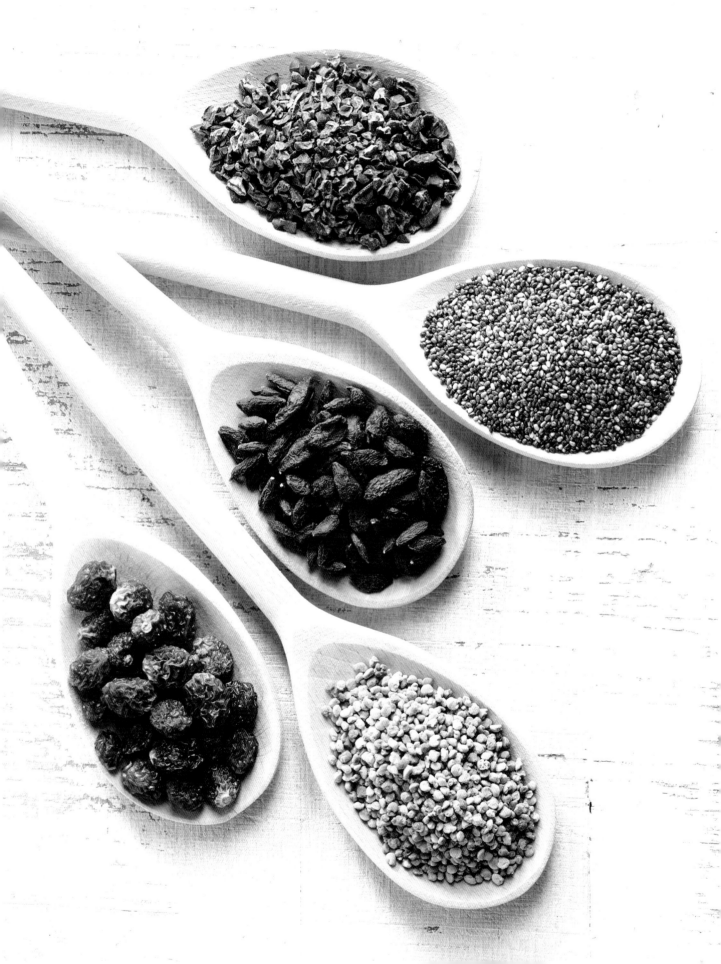

Whole foods mainly include plant-based foods such as vegetables, fruits and nuts, and animal foods such as eggs, meat, fish and poultry.

Whole foods tend to contain high concentrations of antioxidant phenolics, fibre and numerous other phytochemicals that may protect against chronic diseases.

Cacao powder vs cocoa powder

Raw cacao powder is classified a superfood. It is made by cold-pressing unroasted cocoa beans so that the live enzymes in the cacao are retained but the cacao butter (the fat content) is removed, leaving a pure powder.

Cocoa powder might look the same, but it's not! Cocoa is the original cacao powder that has been roasted using very high temperatures. Once this roasting occurs the molecular structure of the cocoa bean changes and the enzyme content is reduced, lowering the overall nutritional and antioxidant value. Refined sugar is often also added to the cocoa powder as part of the sweetening process. It is no longer a superfood.

The secret to healthy chocolate is keeping it raw. Raw cacao powder is high in resveratrol, a polyphenol thought to have antioxidant properties, as well as rich in minerals. Raw cacao can also increase levels of certain neurotransmitters that promote a sense of well-being.

Raw cacao butter also provides these benefits and more, and is also a great source of omega-3 and omega-6 essential fatty acids.

Dairy facts

Do we really need to consume dairy products anymore, now that we have easy access to nut milks, cacao and coconut products?

Much of what we know about milk and dairy produce has been fed to us from the dairy industry – hardly an unbiased view!

If you look at cow's milk with an impartial eye, you'll see that cow's milk, both regular and organic, contains 59 active hormones and scores of allergens, as well as animal-based saturated fat, which includes the animal's cholesterol.

Dairy production is also cruel to animals. A female cow is forced to birth one calf after another, without rest. Calves are taken from their mothers within 12-24 hours of birth so the mother's milk can be used for commercial purposes.

Mother cows, like most mammals, have a strong maternal bond. One study found that this bond was formed in as little as five minutes. When calves are removed, mother cows will frantically bellow for the offspring that they will never see again. Separated calves appear frightened and bewildered.

The calf cannot survive without its mother's milk, so it is taken to slaughter.

To continue producing milk for human consumption, a dairy cow must produce a calf each year.

To keep this trillion dollar industry afloat, cows are fed hormones and a variety of antibiotics to survive reproduction and milk processing. Once taken from the animal, the milk is pasteurised and chemically treated with hormones and antibiotics in order to make it commercially viable. Ingesting such processed food comes at a price. That price is your health.

Dairy is known to be mucous forming and clogging in the body. Most people are lactose intolerant and this difficulty in digesting dairy puts enormous stress on the body, causing a myriad of digestive issues and allergies. Dairy suppresses immune function and is taxing on our bodily organs. Additionally, it offers no real health or environmental advantage at all.

Simply put: humans are designed to drink 'their' mother's milk and calves are designed to drink 'their' mother's milk. We were never meant to swap. This was not nature's intention.

If you remove dairy from your diet, where will you get your calcium from?

Good sources of plant-based calcium include almonds, brazil nuts, sesame seeds, broccoli, bok choy, avocado, coconut meat, pumpkin seeds, flax seeds, collards, okra, spinach, kale, dandelion greens, fennel, cabbage, kidney beans, edamame and asparagus.

Because of the calcium-magnesium ratio in dairy products, our bodies do not properly absorb the calcium it contains. Excess stores of calcium accumulate in our blood and urine and can cause kidney problems, kidney failure or kidney and gall stones. For this reason, plant-based calcium is better assimilated and utilised by the body than calcium found in animal products.

The soy ploy

Soy has been touted as a health food for decades. It was especially popular with vegans and vegetarians as a replacement for dairy, but most soy these days is genetically modified.

Soy may also contain naturally occurring toxins that have been linked to digestive problems, thyroid dysfunction, cognitive decline, reproductive disorders and even heart disease.

If you drink soy milk, consider moving to coconut or

> ### Take note
>
> Both coconut cream and coconut milk make excellent substitutes for dairy products. If you're lactose intolerant or have dairy allergy, you can make use of these foods in your daily cooking just as you would dairy milk or cream.

almond milk for your latte instead.

Fermented soy such as tempeh and miso paste have supposedly kept their health benefits. If you can be sure that your soy products have been locally and organically produced, this might be a safer option. But most soy products have been excessively processed, and this brings its own health risks.

Fermented foods

Fermented foods are pungent, probiotic powerhouses which boost the good bacteria in your digestive tract. Probiotics found naturally in fermented foods are an important part of our diet, because to keep our digestion and immune system strong we must continuously replenish the good bacteria in our gut and digestive tract. This allows us to absorb food nutrients, keep our immune system strong and keep viral, fungal and bacterial infections at bay.

Fermentation is a process of lacto-fermentation in which natural bacteria feed on the sugars and starches in food, creating lactic acid. This process preserves the food, creating beneficial enzymes, vitamins, fatty acids, and various strains of probiotics.

Health experts often recommend fermented foods for gut health. Natural fermentation of foods has also been shown to preserve the nutrients in food and break it down to a more digestible form. This, along with a group of beneficial probiotics created during the fermentation process, could explain the link between consumption of fermented foods and improved digestion.

Coconut vinegar is a wonderful fermented food with good probiotic benefits. Coconut nectar is fermented and then aged naturally for a period of 8-12 months, producing strong pre- and pro-biotic benefits. And it tastes good.

When I drink my coconut vinegar as a shot I literally feel the cleansing effect throughout my body. Coconut vinegar is also delightful as a salad dressing and you will see it being used in a number of recipes throughout this book.

Coconut yoghurt is another good source of probiotics, and a delicious, dairy-free way to work plenty of enzymes and probiotics into your diet.

You can also add some miso, kombucha or sauerkraut to a meal for a good boost of probiotics.

Coconut oil is a powerful anti-bacterial, known for its ability to kill off bad bacteria to avoid overgrowth. Fermented food with natural probiotics will complement this process by replenishing the good bacteria, allowing the body to maintain optimal health through this natural balance.

Gluten-free

Gluten is a protein composite found in foods processed from wheat and related grains such as rye, barley, spelt, triticale and oats. It is used to bind food together and is what gives bread its lovely, chewable texture and makes food thick and tasty.

If you have gluten sensitivities it can be harsh on the immune and digestive system. If you have coeliac disease, the symptoms can be wide-ranging, from mild to severe digestive issues. This problem has become so common that gluten-free diets have become very popular.

However, it's important to watch out for 'gluten-free marketing'. Just because a label claims a product is gluten-free, does not mean that it's not full of sugar, preservatives and other artificial additives, which can be just as bad, if not worse than gluten.

Without gluten to bind food together, food manufacturers often use more (unhealthy) fat and sugar to make the product more palatable, which brings me to the importance of reading labels (see section on page 42).

If you skip the gluten-free ploys and focus on fruits, vegetables, legumes and naturally gluten-free grains such as buckwheat, quinoa and amaranth, this can be a very healthy way of eating.

See page 102 and 104 for a few gluten-free bread recipes.

Non GMO foods

GMO refers to any food product that has been altered at the gene level. These modified foods are newcomers to the world's food supply and we do not know the long-term affects. The first crops of altered foods were created by a subsidiary of agribusiness, Monsanto, in 1994.

GMO foods today include varieties of the soybean, cotton, corn and sugar beets. Grocery manufacturers in the United States estimate that 75% of processed foods in the USA will contain a genetically modified ingredient.

Coconut is not one of these food ingredients.

While the USA and Canada do not label genetically modified foods, other governments – such as Australia, the European Union, Japan and Malaysia – require that food sellers do.

France and Germany were the first to put a ban on GMO foods/crops. Other European countries that placed bans on the cultivation and sale of GMOs include Austria, Hungary, Greece and Luxembourg.

Essential oils

Essential oils are highly concentrated natural oils extracted from plants, flowers, roots, wood, bark or seeds, and are widely known for their healing and purifying benefits. Because of their powerful antioxidant properties, essential oils have been used for thousands of years in a variety of different applications including soaps, perfumes, aromatherapy, skincare products, as well as in medicinal remedies.

Some recipes in this book will include food-grade essential oils both for eating and using topically for skin and hair.

Reading labels

Reading food labels that contain a long list of ingredients can be daunting, and it shouldn't be. It should be simple. Food is food.

If there are any ingredients listed on a package that you don't understand, any numbers you don't recognise, or foods that you prefer not to eat (such as sugar or bad oils) – walk away.

It's important to know that manufacturers have become very creative at hiding things from us. Hydrogenated, partially hydrogenated and vegetable oils – these are all different terms used for trans fats. There are more than 40 names for Monosodium Glutamate (MSG), one of which is 'natural flavours', so it's tricky.

We can't rely on government regulations today because there are so many loopholes and manufacturers know how to hide unpopular ingredients, chemicals and trans fats in their foods.

Look out for chemical and nasty ingredients in body care products too – make sure you read these labels. And remember the word organic does not always make the ingredient healthy.

(I recommend a fabulous book and app called *The Chemical Maze* which is a must-have if you want to better understand the ingredients listed on food and beauty labels.)

Eating organic

An important part of clean eating is eating organic. Organic food contains more nutrients, antioxidants and minerals than its commercially grown counterparts. Organic food is pure, free from chemical additives and flavour enhancers.

Understandably this can sometimes be a challenge. An organic version of your favourite food may not be available, or may be too expensive. So be organic as much as possible and when you do have to pick and choose, be aware of the 'dirty' and the 'clean' dozen. These are the most and least contaminated foods, when industrially farmed.

All fruits and vegetables, whether organic or non-organic, should be washed well before consuming. Non-organic food may be cleaned in water that has coconut vinegar or apple cider vinegar added to it; this helps to remove some of the chemicals.

The Dirty Dozen

The most contaminated foods by industrial farming:

1. Apple
2. All Berries
3. Grapes
4. Celery
5. Capsicum
6. Peaches
7. Potatoes
8. Spinach
9. Cucumber
10. Tomatoes
11. Pears
12. Nectarines

The Clean Dozen

These fruits and vegetables are the least contaminated from pesticides:

1. Avocado
2. Banana
3. Papaya
4. Peas
5. Mango
6. Pineapple
7. Onion
8. Grapefruit
9. Kiwi Fruit
10. Cantaloupe
11. Asparagus
12. Eggplant

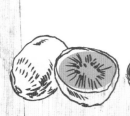
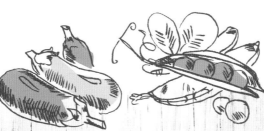
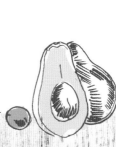

Sustainability and social responsibility

It doesn't make sense to waste food.

When you make almond milk, what do you do with the left-over almond meal? Why not make some bliss balls! I use left-over coconut milk to make a quinoa pudding, or a coconut milk smoothie for breakfast.

Our food from Mother Nature is precious. She provides for us, so let's love, respect and appreciate her.

Eating a plant-based diet also creates lots of food waste. Sometimes after a busy week when I haven't been home much, and there are lots of vegetables left in the fridge, I just juice them all up. It always tastes great!

I also like to compost and put what I can't use or reuse back into the earth.

Buying local as much as possible will help your communities. I buy all of my organic fruit and vegetables from our local organic markets and we get a delivery once a week from our lovely friends at Munch Crunch Organics. I don't always know what's coming but I always like the surprise. This also makes me get creative with recipes, to use up what we've got.

Not all products can be sourced locally however. Our coconut products are produced in Asia and are imported. We support farmers and economy in countries like Thailand, Indonesia and Sri Lanka. We work very closely with our international trade partners to support and develop their growth, their economy, fair trade and sustainable practices.

I visit our suppliers and farms often, and I love experiencing and learning about their culture, and witnessing first-hand their traditional coconut customs, many of which have been practised for generations. It is a gift to be a part of this.

There is no coconut economy in Australia because our growers aren't large enough, and the industry is not yet sustainable enough to match current supply and demand. This may change in time, but will probably take up to 10 years or more. So we will continue to rely on the tropical countries to produce coconuts for our coconut products.

The same applies for other wonderful superfood products, such as maca powder, cacao products, acai and so on, which are all sourced from their originating countries.

When buying imported foods, I can't stress enough the importance of organic. With this certification, you have some guarantee that manufacturing and product standards have been met. It's also important that the importing company has established some fair trade business ethics and practices.

(Our Coconut Magic Raw Energy Bars are made locally in Australia using local and imported ingredients.)

It's your health that matters

I am not one to preach any particular diet, or one single way of eating. I believe that too much rigidity and control may be worse for your health. I personally choose to eat a plant-based diet. I don't eat dairy, poultry or any animal meat. That works for me. I don't think there is one kind of diet that works for all. I'm just saying: include plenty of virgin coconut oil.

To heal or to cleanse your body, live foods, good fats and vegetables usually do the job. If you're embarking on the Candida Cleanse program (see page 56), it's a good idea to maintain a vegan diet, totally meat and dairy free, for a period of time to help minimise acid intake and to rebalance the acid/alkaline pH in your body. Taking a good break will give your body time to cleanse.

MAKE THE SWITCH

Health

Margarine and butter	⇨	Coconut oil, coconut butter, nut butters
Refined cooking oils	⇨	Coconut oil
Refined or processed sugars	⇨	Coconut nectar and coconut sugar
Energy or sports drinks	⇨	Coconut water
Wheat and gluten based grains	⇨	Coconut flour, buckwheat, quinoa (seed)
Soy sauces	⇨	Shoyu nama, coconut aminos, gluten-free tamari
Synthetic protein powders	⇨	Coconut protein powder
Cow's milk	⇨	Coconut milk, nut milk, hempseed milk
Processed chocolate and cocoa	⇨	Raw chocolate, raw cacao
Regular vinegars	⇨	Coconut vinegar

Beauty

Skin lotions	⇨	Coconut oil and cacao butter
Face cleanser	⇨	Coconut oil
Lip balm	⇨	Coconut oil
Hair treatment	⇨	Coconut oil
Oral cleanser	⇨	Coconut oil
Shaving cream	⇨	Coconut oil
Cuticle cream	⇨	Coconut oil

See page 226 for Deodorant and Toothpaste recipes.

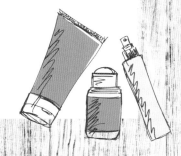

COCONUT OIL FOR DETOX AND ENERGY

We all want more energy, and that's relatively easy to achieve with coconut oil.

If you are used to living a toxic lifestyle, eating processed foods, refined sugars and hydrogenated oils, when you start consuming coconut oil good energy will come, but you may have to go through some detox symptoms first. Thankfully this will only last for a few days.

Coconut oil for the liver

The liver performs many essential functions related to digestion, metabolism, immunity, elimination and the storage of nutrients within the body. These functions make the liver a vital organ; without it, the tissues of the body would quickly die from lack of energy and nutrients.

The liver is considered a gland – an organ that secretes chemicals – because it produces bile, a substance needed to digest fats. Bile salts break up fat into smaller pieces so the fat can be absorbed more easily in the small intestine.

The oil from coconuts is made up of Medium Chain Fatty Acids (MCFAs). Basically, they are smaller fats that are more easily used by your body. Other fats are generally Long Chain Fatty Acids (LCFAs) and are harder to digest.

Bile is not required to break down the MCFAs found in coconut oil, so coconut oil is said to be easy on the liver. This is great for those with NASH (nonalcoholic steatohepatitis), fatty liver, cirrhosis, or any stage of liver disease.

There is no work for the liver and gall bladder to do when digesting MCFAs – so you get an instant energy boost, an increased metabolic rate and subsequently more heat production as well as increased circulation. Coconut oil is therefore an instant source of energy for your body. It's like putting high-octane fuel into your car. And best of all, coconut oil is not stored by the liver as fat in the body.

Detox and antioxidant benefits

Toxic overload in the body can result in a sluggish liver and a lack of energy. Therefore it's important to detox and keep your liver happy.

As metabolism increases so does the body's natural mechanism of detoxification, repair and growth. Even the immune system is shifted to a higher level of efficiency.

The MCFAs in coconut oil destroy disease-causing bacteria, viruses, fungi and parasites. These microorganisms not only cause infection but also often produce toxic byproducts that are carcinogenic or poisonous.

Coconut oil is chemically very stable so it functions as an antioxidant, protecting against destructive free radicals that are often generated by toxins.

Blood sugar balance

Energy comes from glucose from the food we eat. Since glucose is comprised of many long molecule structures, it needs insulin to be able to enter the cells of the body.

The MCFAs in coconut oil (C6-12) are smaller and lighter than glucose, so they can penetrate the cells without the help of insulin. This means that coconut oil can help steady the release of insulin in the body, and help manage those blood sugar spikes from foods containing glucose and fructose.

Whether you have less insulin or insulin resistance, coconut oil still works. You can take coconut oil to improve the function of your pancreas and/or activate your insulin response.

HEALTHY FATS FOR HEALTHY WEIGHT

While offering people an experience of our coconut oil, many people (particularly women) ask me: won't this make me fat?

I always respond with a resounding NO. Coconut oil will not store in your body as fat, and it therefore will not contribute to weight gain. How wonderful is that!

And not only will coconut oil not store in the body as fat, it will actually help your liver and metabolism work more effectively. This allows your body to naturally shed excess weight and, thanks to coconut oil's stabilising effect, the body can return to its natural healthy weight.

MCFAs and oil blends containing MCFAs have received considerable attention recently for their ability to reduce abdominal obesity and diminish fat storage in the body. Coconut oil has been proven to have fat-burning effects (known as thermogenesis). Some body-builders use coconut oil to help metabolise fat. So if you are trying to lose weight, this can be a good boost!

Dr Raymond Peat, a leading researcher in the field of hormones, tells a story about how farmers in the 1940s attempted to use coconut oil to fatten their animals, but unexpectedly, they found it made their animals lean and active. This was not the result they were hoping for, as they wanted to fatten their animals in preparation for slaughter. They then switched to using soy and corn feed. Soy and corn feed slows down the thyroid, causing animals to get fat without eating much food.

For a more human example: when I was presenting at a trade show a few years ago, a very excited and energetic woman shared with me her experience of coconut oil. She had been taking just one teaspoon each morning over a few months, and had lost much of the weight around her hips and waist. This was stubborn, unmovable weight that she had tried and tried to lose. I think her excitement came both from having lost the weight and from having kept it off, one year later.

So why is coconut oil the fat that makes you thin?

Coconut oil is a medium chain fat that is processed by the liver and is converted directly into energy. This gives the liver a powerful boost which helps the process of elimination, and gives your metabolism a boost as well. When the liver and metabolism are working effectively, the body has plenty of available energy to burn, and that's what happens to the kilojoules consumed. They are burned off rather than stored. This allows excess body fat to naturally drop off.

Coconut oil also assists weight loss because it is known to curb cravings, and many detox specialists advise their clients to take a teaspoon of coconut oil when they crave either sugar or carbohydrates. A craving is an imbalance in the body, and coconut oil helps to rebalance the system.

Recipes for energy and to assist with weight loss

✓ Coconut Lemon Detox, page 84

✓ Beautiful Skin Smoothie, page 81

✓ Green Detox Soup, page 124

✓ Green Mint Tea, page 84

Weight loss tip

Studies show that after eating a meal that contains medium chain triglycerides (MCTs) your metabolism increases by up to 48%. This helps burn up the kilojoules consumed in that meal. If you're using coconut oil to lose weight, take one tablespoon three times per day, before or with each meal. Or use the equivalent amount in your cooking.

COCONUT OIL AND COCONUT FOR HEALTH

Can you still get all of the amazing benefits of the coconut by eating the flesh, drinking coconut water, or coconut milk? Yes!

Everything coconut is healthy and beneficial, however coconut oil contains a concentrated dose of the healing properties of lauric, capric and caprylic acid – nature's anti-bacterial, anti-viral and anti-fungal magic!

Coconut water

Coconut water is an excellent source of hydration, electrolytes and minerals. It's known as nature's sports drink, and is rich in potassium, sodium and energy-producing carbohydrates.

Researchers have found that coconut water is more effective than a traditional sports drink in maintaining hydration and promoting recovery between work-out sessions. An even bigger bonus is that unprocessed coconut water is free of the artificial colours, flavours and preservatives found in most commercial sports drinks.

The best coconut water to drink is straight from the coconut within hours of it coming off the tree. If you're not living in a tropical climate, however, that might not be possible.

Coconut water has gained enormous popularity in the past few years and there are now many brands on the market, many of which have been pasteurised or preserved. This is done so coconut water can maintain some shelf life – sadly it also kills off all of the sensitive enzymes and minerals and therefore reduces the health benefits.

If you can't get your coconut water from a fresh coconut then try to stick with an organic or reputable brand. It is best to avoid aluminium tins, as these are often sterilised with chemicals - and they leach.

Coconut meat

Coconut meat is a great source of roughage if you are having trouble going! If you are undertaking a healing fast, as recommended by Dr Bruce Fife in his book, *Coconut Cures*, you can add a small handful of coconut meat to your food each day, to provide the required roughage to keep you regular. (This was a good alternative for me when I was doing his fast).

Healthy digestion and nutrient absorption

Most Naturopaths or health practitioners will tell you that in order to heal your body, you need to heal your digestion.

This is because up to 80% of our immune system lives in the digestive tract. The digestive process is vital for nutrient absorption, hormone balance, blood sugar balance, waste elimination and weight loss. Practically every part of the human bodily function is connected to this system.

Part of the reason I became sick in Thailand was because my digestion was so weak. My immune system crashed and my whole body became vulnerable. Having a weak digestive system can lead to a horrible downward spiral.

Coconut oil strengthens and supports digestion in the following ways:

- Its anti-microbial properties benefit intestinal health by killing troublesome microorganisms that may cause chronic inflammation.

- Because it slows digestion, coconut oil also helps prevent blood sugar fluctuations after a meal by slowing the rate carbohydrates are broken down into blood glucose.

- When the digestion of food is slowed down, it helps you to feel fuller after a meal. Many people notice that after adding coconut oil to their diet, they are less prone to snacking.

- The medium-chain fatty acids in coconut oil destroy candida, a condition of yeast overgrowth in the body, which triggers symptoms of weight gain, carbohydrate cravings, fatigue and many other conditions. Eliminating candida is an important part of achieving permanent weight loss.

- Coconut oil is excellent for detoxification. It cleanses the body of many infirmities, balances the digestive tract and nourishes all cells in the body. These benefits restore your health and pave the way again for healthy weight management.

- People who suffer from malabsorption problems such as cystic fibrosis, and have difficulty digesting or absorbing fats and fat soluble vitamins, benefit greatly from MCFAs. They can also be of importance for people suffering from diabetes, obesity, gall bladder disease, pancreatitis, Crohn's disease, pancreatic insufficiency, and some forms of cancer.

- As we get older our bodies don't function as well as they did in earlier years. Our pancreas doesn't make as many digestive enzymes, our intestines don't absorb nutrients as well, and the whole process of digestion and elimination moves at a less efficient rate. As a result, older people often suffer from vitamin and mineral deficiencies. Because MCFAs are easy to digest and improve vitamin and mineral absorption, they should be included in meals for older people. This is easy to do if the meals are prepared with coconut oil.

Coconut oil has become a lifesaver for many people, particularly the very young and the very old, and for those who suffer digestive disorders and have trouble digesting fats. For the same reason, it is also used in infant formula for the treatment of malnutrition.

Try these recipes for healthy digestion:

✔ Belly Soother Smoothie, page 80

✔ Chai Spice Smoothie, page 80

✔ Young Coconut Soup, page 128

Curb sugar and carbohydrate cravings

A craving is your body's way of saying it needs something. The need then filters through the mind and the habitual memory kicks in of that lovely sweet burst of simple sugar energy. What the body really wants to say (without the interference of the mind) is: 'I need some nutrition!'

Because MCFAs in coconut oil go straight to your liver to be used as energy, coconut oil is a source of instant energy for your body, much like sugar and simple carbohydrates. But unlike carbs and simple sugars, coconut oil delivers quick energy without producing an insulin spike in your bloodstream. This means there is no energy slump afterwards, and this in turn curbs that craving for an energy fix.

Eat a tablespoon of coconut oil to kill cravings immediately!

BRAIN HEALTH

Alzheimer's Disease currently affects 5.2 million people in the U.S. and is the seventh leading cause of death in that country. The cost of treating it is estimated at USD$148 billion.

There are more than 342,800 Australians living with dementia. Each week there are more than 1,800 new cases of dementia in Australia. That means approximately one person every six minutes is diagnosed. Did you know that coconut oil has a role to play in preventing, slowing and reversing this disease?

Dr Mary Newport, MD, treated her husband with coconut oil and MCT oil, with amazing results.

In 2003, at the age of 53, Steve Newport began showing signs of progressive dementia. At that time, his wife was medical director of the neonatal intensive care unit at Spring Hill Regional Hospital in Florida.

Brain boosting foods

- ✔ Coconut Oil
- ✔ Avocado
- ✔ Blueberries
- ✔ Cacao
- ✔ Bananas
- ✔ Hempseeds
- ✔ Leafy Greens
- ✔ Nuts/Activated Nuts
- ✔ Chia seeds

He was given Alzheimer's drugs but the disease steadily worsened, and he was experiencing side effects from the drugs. (It should be noted that the latest research shows that the various Alzheimer's drugs, like Aricept, have proven to be disappointing, with little real benefit and often distressing side effects.)

When Dr Newport couldn't get her husband into a drug trial for a new Alzheimer's medication, she started researching the mechanism behind the disease. She discovered that certain brain cells may have difficulty utilising glucose (which is made from the carbohydrates we eat) and when this happens, precious neurons begin to die.

Research led her to discover an alternative energy source for brain cells – fats known as ketones. Under certain conditions (for example, in a low carbohydrate diet) MCTs are converted by the liver into ketones. (In the first few weeks of life, ketones provide about 25% of the energy newborn babies need to survive.)

Dr Newport learned that the ingredient in the drug trial was a synthetic version of MCT oil, derived from coconut or palm kernel oil, at a dose of 20 g (about 20 ml or 4 teaspoons) per day.

According to the latest research, when MCT oil is metabolised, the ketones which the body creates not only protect against the incidence of Alzheimer's, but may actually reverse it.

So she began giving Steve coconut oil, twice a day. At this point, he could barely remember how to draw a clock. Two weeks after adding coconut oil to his diet, his drawing improved. After 37 days, Steve's drawing gained even more clarity.

The oil seemed to lift the fog, and in the first 60 days, Dr Newport saw remarkable changes in him.

Over the next year, the dementia continued to reverse itself: Steve was able to run again, his reading comprehension improved dramatically, and his short-term memory was improving. An MRI test also showed that the brain atrophy had been completely halted.

It's enough to make a drug company start worrying about its future monopoly and long-term profits.

For more information, see Dr Newport's on her husband's recovery video uploaded by the IHMC and Tedx Talks on YouTube.

Dr Newport has also written a book on her research: *Alzheimer's Disease, what if there was a cure?*

Sadly, you will not find any information on ketones, or the use of coconut oil or MCT oil, on any Alzheimer's Association websites.

Recipes for brain health:

✔ Creamy Berry Magic Smoothie, page 82

✔ Berry Bliss Bars, page 218

✔ Avocado and Coconut Popsicles, page 224

✔ All Desserts, page 208

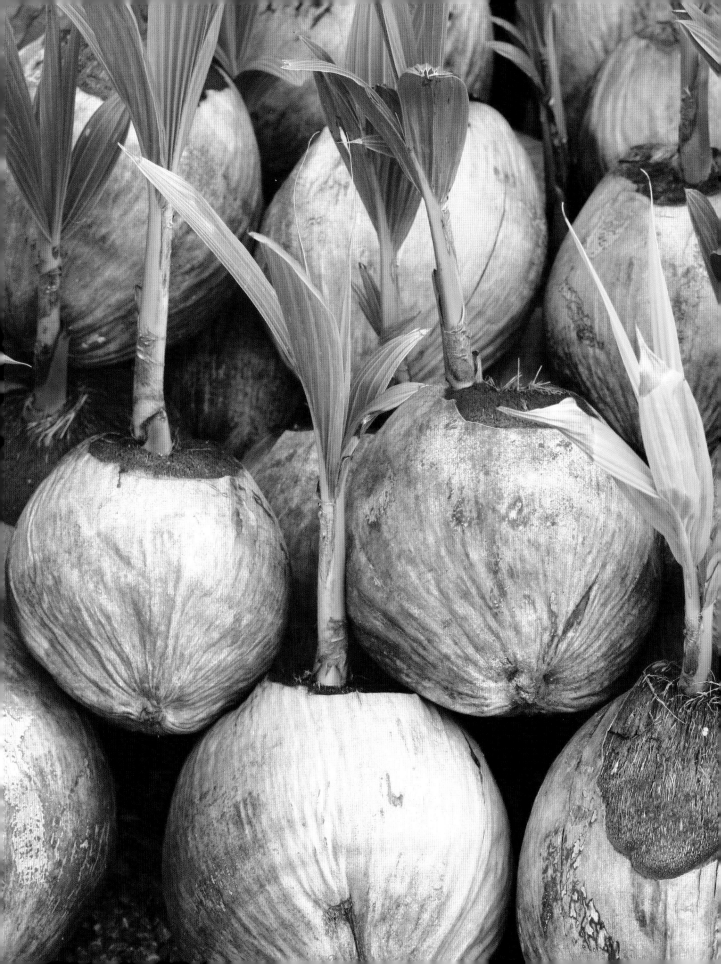

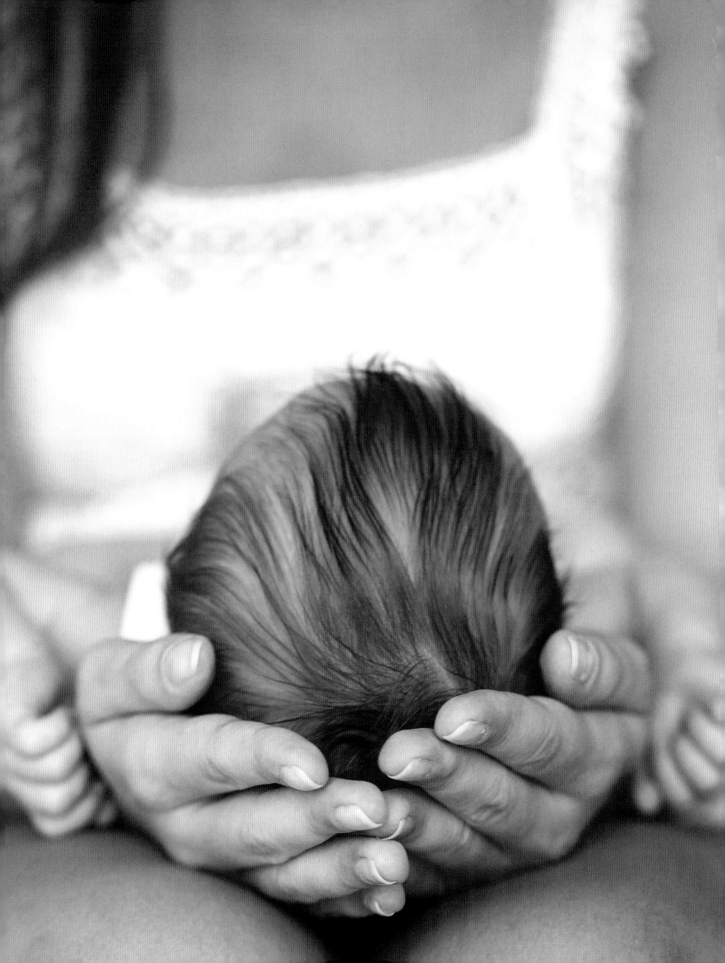

PREGNANCY AND BABY CARE

We all want to have a happy and healthy pregnancy. We all want to be sure that we're giving our body and our babies the best possible nourishment during and after gestation.

Coconut oil has some remarkable benefits when it comes to pregnancy, which is why it's known as the 'Breast Milk of Mother Nature'.

Just as breast milk is jam-packed with nutrients and disease-fighting ingredients to keep baby healthy, so is coconut oil. The lauric acid in coconut oil is a natural way to strengthen your immune system, and that of your baby.

The benefits of coconut oil during and after pregnancy include:

Lactation: Coconut oil stimulates metabolism, promoting both a healthy thyroid and lactation. Intake of coconut oil while pregnant may help ensure a good milk supply. Studies have shown that the milk from breast-feeding mothers who take coconut oil and other coconut products contains a higher amount of lauric acid.

Stretch marks: Because of the high amount of vitamin E in coconut oil, pregnant women in South India apply the coconut extract on their bellies to prevent stretch marks. Even existing stretch marks have a chance to fade with regular use of Coconut Magic coconut oil. It will also moisturise the skin and keep skin irritation and infection at bay.

One of our customers believes that by taking a coconut oil bath two to three times per week during her pregnancy, she had no stretch marks whatsoever. She happily shared this on a Facebook thread. (See recipe on page 226 for bath time fun.)

Infant health: Coconut oil helps develop the immune system of the newborn as well as aiding brain and bone development. It is known to relieve nappy (diaper) rash, Keratosis Pilaris (a common, harmless skin condition), and is gentle and beneficial for baby's digestive health

Pregnancy can be a stressful time, and pregnant women have an increased demand for good nutrition. The unborn child also demands ample nutrients for proper development and growth, and will steal them from the mother's body if they are not supplied in her diet.

For generations people living in the coconut-growing regions of the world have relied on coconut for nature's nourishment and health. Modern medicine has also recognised the health benefits of the MCFAs in coconut oil, which is now used by hospitals in infant formula.

Premature and infants who are ill, especially whose digestive organs are underdeveloped, are able to absorb MCFA with relative ease, while other fats pass through their system pretty much undigested.

Whenever I see pregnant ladies or mums with babies I get very excited about sharing with them the wonderful benefits of coconut oil. Sadly there are companies producing baby products that are toxic and dangerous. In 2011, Johnson & Johnson was sued for selling shampoo and baby wash that allegedly contained methylene chloride, an ingredient used in cosmetics that was banned by the FDA because of its link to cancer. The law firm that filed the suit was also investigating other suspect product ingredients.

Nappy rash cream

There is no risk to the baby's bottom, because coconut oil is pure and contains no added chemicals. With its impressive anti-fungal, anti-bacterial and anti-viral properties, it can even heal yeast infections. As an added bonus coconut oil smells delicious. It will not ruin cloth nappies like many other nappy rash creams do.

Apply a thin layer to the affected area.

Cradle cap

Massage coconut oil onto your baby's scalp and leave for about 20 minutes. The coconut oil will moisturise and nourish baby's scalp and loosen the cradle cap flakes. After 20 minutes wash off the oil, or wipe clean with a damp cloth and gently comb the hair with a soft brush to remove any loose flakes. Regular treatments will keep baby's scalp moistened and nourished and will help prevent cradle cap from re-occurring.

Baby massage oil

The benefits of baby massage are endless. It strengthens the bond between mother and baby, it helps baby to relax and sleep at bedtime. '

Coconut oil is pure and safe as well as nourishing and healing for baby's tender and sensitive skin. The beautiful subtle aroma of coconut is also calming for your baby's senses.

Adding coconut oil and a drop of pure lavender oil will make bath time soothing, moisturising and relaxing for both baby and Mum.

Thrush, yeast and candida

Taken both internally and externally, coconut oil can help treat the yeast that causes thrush and candida. A little coconut oil dabbed inside the baby's mouth and on mum's nipples before breast-feeding is an effective way for baby to receive the benefits. And if mum eats some oil, the benefits are multiplied!

Applying coconut oil to a nursing mum's nipples will also help with painful cracks and irritation.

Teething

Coconut oil is pure and safe to eat therefore it is also safe to pop into the baby's mouth. Rub the oil directly onto the gums of teething babies and children to ease the pain.

HORMONE AND THYROID HEALTH

Hormones are your body's chemical messengers, travelling in your bloodstream to tissues and organs. They work slowly, over time, and affect many different processes, including:

✓ Growth and development

✓ Metabolism – how your body gets energy from the foods you eat

✓ Sexual function

✓ Reproduction

✓ Mood.

Hormones are produced using good fats and cholesterol, so ingesting bad fats, and not enough good fats, can have a detrimental effect on this system.

Coconut oil works wonders for hormone health, providing the necessary building blocks for hormone production. Dr Raymond Peat believes that coconut oil, when taken together with a balanced diet, helps lower cholesterol to normal by assisting its conversion to pregnenolone, the precursor to many hormones, including progesterone. Dr Peat recommends increasing pregnenolone for women with hormone imbalances.

Research points to the fact that an underactive thyroid gland may be the number one cause of weight problems, especially among women. Thyroid hormones are required for normal health and the activity of every cell in the body. It therefore makes sense that a deficiency in these hormones will have a detrimental effect on the entire body.

The thyroid gland is the body's metabolic thermostat, controlling body temperature, energy use and the growth rate in children. If you have a sluggish thyroid, you may lack energy, suffer from depression, weight gain, low body temperature, headaches, menstrual disorders, dry skin, insomnia, puffy eyes, brittle nails, mental dullness, dizziness and a low sex drive.

According to Dr Peat, the sudden surge of polyunsaturated oils into the food chain post World War II has caused many changes in our hormones. These polyunsaturated oils interfere with the thyroid gland and block the secretion of this hormone.

Unrefined virgin coconut oil does not inhibit thyroid function in the way that these unsaturated vegetable oils do. Because of its effect on metabolism and energy in the body, consuming coconut oil regularly is known to help restore thyroid function.

I have met women who have lost weight by taking coconut oil daily, bringing their hormones back into balance. They then use Coconut Magic coconut oil on their bodies to avoid any 'saggy skin' caused by rapid weight loss.

Simply switching from hydrogenated unsaturated or refined oils to coconut oil can be enough for you to start experiencing these amazing benefits.

We cannot have proper hormonal balance without adequate amounts of saturated fats. If you really need hormone help, aim to consume 1/4 cup of added coconut oil per day.

Benefits that coconut oil offer for balancing hormones when taken internally, can also help to increase your sex drive.

Hormones are produced using good fats and cholesterol, so a deficiency of these nutrients can cause hormone problems, because the body doesn't have the building blocks to make them.

In 2013 I went to see Dr Gabrielle Cousens at an event in Brisbane. During his presentation he mentioned the benefits of coconut oil as neuro- and cardio-protective, and how it is exceptionally good for treating Alzheimer's disease. He explained that the fat is converted directly by the liver into ketones which go right through to the brain and energise it. This is because the brain is made of 70-80% saturated fat.

He also said that coconut oil would raise good cholesterol, for women in particular, and that this would also support the thyroid, and also hormone production.

Intrigued, I went to see a local GP for blood tests. Sure enough, Dr Cousens was right. My LDL cholesterol was normal and my HDL was high, this being a sign of good health and balanced hormone production.

THE CANDIDA CLEANSE

What you can do

When candida proliferates in the body, it means the balance between good and bad bacteria is lost, and the bad bacteria have proliferated. The solution is:

1. Kill off some of the bad bacteria with coconut oil

2. Starve the overgrowth by eliminating sugars, dairy, yeast and grains from the diet; this stops feeding the growth of bad bacteria

3. Feed the good bacteria so it can regain control. This includes taking a good probiotic

4. Build the body's immune system so its natural defenses can step up

5. Balance the body's pH by alkalising the system. (There are an abundance of food plans for alkalising the body – Google 'alkaline foods')

Here's what I did over a four-week period. I call it the Candida Cleanse.

Disclaimer: Please check with your Naturopath or health physician before you attempt this diet. I am not a qualified health practitioner – I am simply sharing what worked for me. This Cleanse is based on information from Dr Fife's book, Coconut Cures.

Weeks one and two

Each day I took three tablespoons of coconut oil. I drank one to two litres of water, with plenty of lemon juice – this helped to wash the coconut oil down. I drank one anti-candida smoothie per day. (Recipe on page 80.)

The lemon juice helped alkalise my body and balance the

pH; the coconut oil and anti-candida drink (which also has coconut oil in it) kills off the bad bacteria.

I didn't have access to a quality source of probiotics so I learned to make my own cashew and coconut yoghurts, (recipe on page 112) and used this as a daily internal probiotic. I also drank rejuvelac (a fermented beverage that is inexpensive, easy to make and full of wonderful nutrients for your body) and fermented sauerkraut daily.

I applied coconut oil to my skin topically. This is also deeply absorbed by the body and helps build the skin's natural immune system.

I avoided refined sugars, wheat, dairy, yeast and grains.

I still had some low sugar fruits, such as grapefruit and papaya. This kept me sane, and alkalised. The papaya is also a great belly soother.

I took some ginger infused in warm water to help settle the bouts of nausea, especially in the initial days during the healing crisis.

For week two, repeat week one, but increase your daily dose of coconut oil to five tablespoons per day.

(Optional) Week three – The Coconut Oil Detox

The coconut oil detox is designed to aid chronic gut infections and digestive problems. It is designed to flush out candida and any other organisms that have overstayed their welcome. I recommend if you are going to do the one week fast that you make it a time that you can relax and have time out without the pressures of work or family commitments. If this is not possible, maintain the diet as recommended in weeks one and two, whilst continuing to increase your coconut oil dose each day.

I stopped all food except for the cashew yoghurt and coconut oil. I also included fresh coconut water (one coconut) each day, and a handful of coconut meat for fibre. I increased my daily dose of coconut oil to 10 tablespoons per day.

In his book, *Coconut Cures*, Dr Bruce Fife recommends up to 15 tablespoons per day of coconut oil during the coconut oil detox. I found that 10 was my body's limit.

It is also recommended to do this fast for a minimum of three days. The initial days may promote a healing crisis, which is normal as the good bacteria goes to war with the bad. I fasted like this, on the coconut oil detox, for seven days.

Week Four

This is the same as Week Two.

After four weeks of building the good bacteria and killing off the bad I was fully healthy again, with clear skin, stronger digestion and much better energy levels. From this point I started to re-introduce my favourite fruits, such as pineapple and mangos, grains and sugar-free desserts (using coconut or natural sweeteners).

To this day I continue to eat coconut oil and probiotic-rich foods such as coconut cider vinegar, fermented sauerkraut and miso to help maintain the balance in my system.

I also recommend a diet high in raw foods to assist with the detox. Go for one raw meal per day, and one green anti-candida smoothie per day.

Be sure to include:

✓ Coconut and cashew yoghurt

✓ Coconut vinegar shots

✓ Fermented foods such as sauerkraut

✓ Therapeutic daily dose of coconut oil

✓ No refined sugars or yeast

✓ Stay alkaline with lemon water/ginger water blends.

Recipes for the Candida Cleanse

✓ The Anti-Candida drink, page 80
✓ Cashew Yoghurt, page 112
✓ Fresh salad from the Super Salads recipe section.

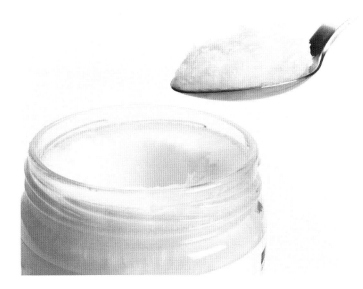

OIL PULLING THERAPY

This is by far the number one health tip for using coconut oil. Oil Pulling Therapy deserves so much attention!

Oil pulling is an ancient Ayurvedic health tradition for detoxification and rejuvenation of the entire system. This simple morning practice offers remarkable results.

Stories abound on the internet about the introduction of oil pulling to the west by a Dr Karach. We were unable to find any biographical evidence of Dr Karach, (but see www.oilpulling.com) however the benefits of oil pulling speak for themselves.

Dr Karach claimed that oil pulling could help a variety of illnesses ranging from heart disease and digestive troubles to hormonal disorders. Apparently he used the method in his medical practice with great success. He said it helped him recover from a chronic blood disorder and arthritis, which at times was so painful he was bedridden.

Traditionally, oil pullers used sesame or sunflower oil. Today virgin coconut oil is the preferred choice, as it offers the additional benefits of anti-microbial, anti-fungal, anti-inflammatory, anti-bacterial and enzymatic properties. Coconut oil also helps to remove plaque from your teeth and it also strengthens gums by thoroughly cleansing the gum line.

The best time to oil pull is first thing in the morning on an empty stomach, as your body is in its natural detox mode. Simply put one tablespoon of coconut oil in your mouth and swish it around for 15-20 minutes, just as you would a regular mouthwash. In the first 5 minutes the mouth cleansing effects will occur, as you reach 10 minutes, the fat enzymes in the oil will start to 'pull' the pus, toxins and bacteria from your body and the detox benefits begin to occur.

Once you've finished swishing, spit out the oil into a bin (not down the sink). Do not swallow, as this is now toxic.

Brush your teeth and give your mouth a good clean. If you use a mild flavoured coconut oil it is quite pleasant. If it is cold and the oil is solid, it will only take a minute for it to melt inside your mouth.

Whilst you are swishing the oil in your mouth the fat enzymes in the oil literally 'pull' congestion and mucus from your throat and loosen up your sinuses. The process removes bacteria, toxins and parasites that live in your mouth or lymph system. Dr Fife uses the following analogy. 'It acts much like the oil you put in your car engine. The oil picks up dirt and grime. When you drain the oil, it pulls out the dirt and grime with it, leaving the engine relatively clean. Consequently, the engine runs smoother and lasts longer. Likewise, when we expel harmful substances from our bodies our health is improved and we run smoother and last longer.'

Detoxifying the Body Through Oral Cleansing

After coming across the work of the Weston A Price foundation and Dr Bruce Fife and the many success stories related to the therapy, I decided to try it for myself.

Before oil pulling I had a particular problem tooth, which caused nerve pain and sensitivity for at least one year. Dentists wanted to do a root canal, but I refused. Since oil pulling my overall dental health has improved dramatically, and I have had no teeth or gum problems.

I also used to get acne blemishes, but after the first month of oil pulling I had no breakouts at all! It made my skin clear and smooth again. I learnt that the therapy cleanses bacteria from the body and also helps to balance hormones. It has helped with period cramps, digestion, immunity, and PMS symptoms. Plus, the more subtle benefits of oil pulling include an overall improved sense of well-being: I have more energy and I feel lighter and clearer in my mind.

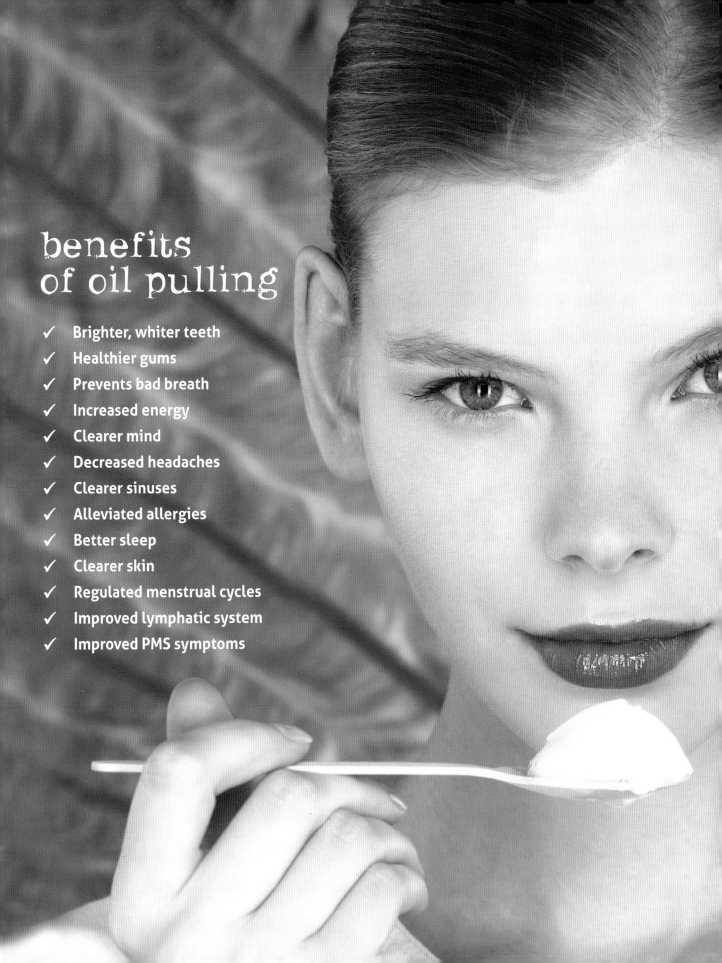

benefits
of oil pulling

- ✓ **Brighter, whiter teeth**
- ✓ **Healthier gums**
- ✓ **Prevents bad breath**
- ✓ **Increased energy**
- ✓ **Clearer mind**
- ✓ **Decreased headaches**
- ✓ **Clearer sinuses**
- ✓ **Alleviated allergies**
- ✓ **Better sleep**
- ✓ **Clearer skin**
- ✓ **Regulated menstrual cycles**
- ✓ **Improved lymphatic system**
- ✓ **Improved PMS symptoms**

COCONUT OIL FOR HEALING

Something's in the air, and mostly it's not good for us.

The air we breathe and the food we eat is heavily contaminated by harmful chemicals and other toxic substances. These are known as environmental toxins and are impossible to avoid. They include:

- PCBs (polychlorinated biphenyls), an industrial chemical that has been banned in the United States for decades, yet is a persistent organic pollutant that's still present in our environment

- Pesticides that are sprayed on our food and end up in our water supply

- Mould and other fungal toxins that are present in buildings; in foods such as peanuts, wheat, corn and alcoholic drinks

- Phthalates, chemicals that are used to increase the life of fragrances and soften plastics

- VOCs (Volatile Organic Compounds) that are found in our drinking water, in our carpets and in paints, and in deodorants and cleaning fluids

- Dioxins, which are chemical compounds formed from commercial waste incineration and from burning fuels. Dioxins are found in animal fats

- Asbestos, which was widely used for insulating buildings in the 1950s and 60s

Coconut oil protection

Coconut oil is ideal for creating the protective layers we need to counter environmental toxins. Apply liberally to the skin daily after a shower, or in the shower, to build your skin's natural immune system.

Skin tissue damage

Skin tissue damage is caused by a variety of factors – sun exposure, environmental pollution, dehydration, cigarette smoke, poor diet and lack of exercise – but more recent evidence points to the rise of free radicals in our bodies.

Free radicals are oxygen molecules that have become unstable and reactive; they are 'free' because they are missing a critical molecule, and so off they go, hunting for another molecule to pair with. They bounce around cells and tissues, depleting healthy molecules and causing damage, not just to one molecule, but to many, setting off a chain reaction.

When a free radical oxidises a fatty acid, it changes that fatty acid into a free radical, which then damages another fatty acid...and so on...

These attacks can overwhelm the body's natural free-radical defence system, and the damage can lead to a host of chronic diseases. It is now believed that free radicals are the primary cause of ageing, as this damage often becomes visible on our skin as wrinkles, blemishes, age spots, liver spots and lingering scars.

The largest source of free radicals comes from cooked, rancid and oxidised oils – mainly polyunsaturated vegetable oils – used commercially in food manufacturing. These oils, soy products and margarines are rancid and toxic because of the way they are produced, even before they are added to manufactured foods.

Other oils such as flax, olive, hemp, nut and seed oils and so on, are light to moderately stable, but are extremely heat- and light-sensitive and can become oxidised, rancid and even toxic when left exposed to light and/or heat.

When oxidative damage or rancidity occurs, the oil

becomes sticky and can cause damage to brain cells, and can cause inflammation and an increase in the risk of diabetes and cardiovascular disease.

Coconut oil reverses skin tissue damage

Coconut oil as a skin moisturiser has a pleasant odour and provides a beautiful radiance and glow to the skin – but it's the ability of coconut oil to reverse skin tissue damage that sets it apart from other moisturisers.

You can nourish and repair the skin with coconut oil, both externally and internally. Coconut oil reverses the oxidative process by displacing the cooked oil from tissues and providing fat-soluble vitamins, minerals, and super nutrition factors directly to the damaged tissues.

Digestive disorders

Irritable bowel syndrome (IBS), Crohn's disease, candida, acid reflux, constipation, kidney and gallstones are a few of the more common digestive disorders.

Coconut oil as a digestive remedy

Coconut oil may help to improve the digestive system, preventing various stomach and digestion-related problems, including IBS. The MCFAs in coconut oil have anti-microbial properties that help the body fight off bacteria, fungi, parasites and so on, that cause digestive upsets. Coconut oil helps to 'get things working' in the process of elimination and therefore relieves constipation.

According to Dr Bruce Fife in his book *Coconut Cures*, coconut oil:

✓ Relieves symptoms associated with Crohn's disease, IBS, ulcerative colitis, gallbladder disease and stomach ulcers

✓ Expels or kills tapeworms, lice, giardia, and other parasites

✓ Dissolves kidney stones.

Acne therapy

Acne therapy is similar to a face cleansing therapy. Simply wet your face with water, massage just ½ teaspoon of coconut oil into your face and then pat dry with a warm face cloth. This will leave a layer of light oil on your skin to do its magic. Please note that the face has smaller absorption glands than the body and will therefore require much smaller amounts of oil to be applied. Don't overdo it!

Coconut oil also helps in absorption of other nutrients such as vitamins, minerals and amino acids.

Skin wounds, acne, eczema and bruises

I suffered chronic eczema attacks for years, with horrible, red, bumpy and itchy skin, often with no relief. It wasn't until I started to use coconut oil on my body that I found a permanent solution.

Coconut oil for skin health

Coconut oil on its own or as a carrier for essential oils is a great way to treat skin wounds topically. Mixed with Tea Tree oil it has powerful antiseptic, anti-microbial and anti-fungal effects that may help treat fungus overgrowth, open cuts and sores, rashes or skin irritations such as psoriasis, eczema and athlete's foot. When applied on scrapes and cuts, coconut oil forms a thin layer that protects the wound from outside dust, bacteria and viruses.

Coconut oil speeds up the healing process of bruises by repairing damaged tissues.

Lauric acid found in coconut oil has naturally occurring antiseptic properties that can stop the common bacteria associated with acne much better than chemical-laden over-the-counter acne medications.

Coconut oil is a powerful natural anti-fungal, and because it is also gentle and pure, it is also safe to use in treating these conditions for babies and children.

Coconut oil can also help with skin problems such as psoriasis, dermatitis and eczema.

Treating acne with coconut oil

It seems counter-intuitive to consider treating an excess of oil with more oil. However when looking into the science of this it actually does make sense.

Our skin produces a natural oil known as sebum, which is made up of medium chain fatty acids, just as coconut oil is. This oil is secreted by the body through sebum glands located under the skin. Acne is created when skin cells, sebum and hair clump together to form a plug; this plug gets infected with bacteria, resulting in a swelling. A pimple starts to develop when the plug begins to break down.

Coconut oil is anti-bacterial, so when applied to the inflamed sebum gland, or the pimple, it actually helps to reduce the inflammation by killing off the excess bacteria in that gland.

This is why a good quality coconut oil – one that is not blended with cheap or refined oils and therefore maintaining its full MCFA content – will be effective in the reduction of acne.

COCONUT OIL FOR BEAUTY

I started to share my passion for coconut oil on the island of Koh Samui in Thailand, where a good friend of mine remained interested and supportive, but she never bought any for herself.

Fast forward to a few months later: at the end of one of her regular visits she said, 'I'll take one of those one litre bottles of coconut oil.' When I queried why, after so long, she said, 'Because I've seen your skin transform over these past couple of months, and I'm ready to use it for myself.'

Having lived on the islands for a significant period of time, I saw the islanders use coconut oil for many things, particularly for skincare. I discovered that they knew something important about coconut oil.

The Islanders would rise in the morning, wash or shower with soap and water and then coat their skin in coconut oil. They would then go out for the day in the tropical sun. Their skin was not blemished, burnt, scaly or dried out. They looked younger than their western counterparts, often with a beautiful tan. Skin conditions such as eczema, psoriasis and fungal infections were almost unheard of. All of these benefits came because they were replenishing their skin's natural oils with coconut oil.

The MCFAs found in sebum, the body's natural oil, hold natural anti-fungal, anti-bacterial and anti-viral properties that hydrate, heal and rebuild the skin's immune system. After washing, if we replenish with coconut oil we're replacing those natural immune-building and healing properties in a way that our skin's cells can easily absorb and process.

I now use coconut oil in all my beauty routines, and I have replaced all my chemically based cleansers and moisturisers with only the purest, organic coconut oil.

Once I started to read the packages of commercially-bought cosmetics and moisturisers, I realised how much damage these products were doing to my skin.

There are creams for everything: for day, for night, for lips, for eyes, for face, for body, for feet, for hair, for hands, for cuticles, for knees, for elbows. The majority of them contain chemicals and ingredients that were never meant to be applied to the skin.

When it comes to putting things on my body, I follow this general guideline: If you can't eat it, don't put it on your skin.

Would you deliberately eat cetyl alcohol, isopropyl alcohol, ammonium lauryl sulfate, butylated hydroxytoluene, or silicone-derived ingredients such as cyclomethicone? How about polydimethylsiloxane, or diprobase? Sodium lauryl sulfate is used in thousands of cosmetic products, and, ironically, it originates from coconuts, but this chemical is anything but natural. Putting these and other chemicals on your skin or scalp may actually be worse than eating them, because when you do, they are absorbed straight into the bloodstream without filtering of any kind, going directly to delicate organs.

I believe that the key to naturally radiant and glowing skin is to only apply to your skin and body what is completely pure and clean – it's really that simple.

Which oils?

A test of a good quality coconut oil is how well it is absorbed by the skin. A coconut oil with a high concentration of MCFAs will be rapidly taken up by the skin, because the body recognises it is getting quality hydration. MCFAs

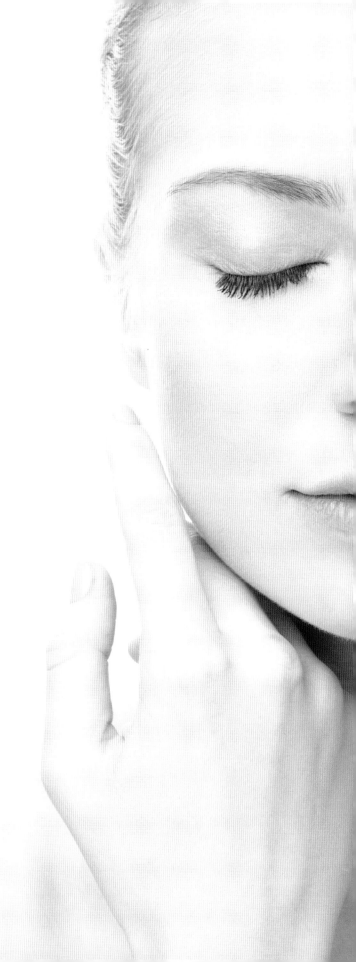

are easily absorbed by the skin and do not leave a thick residue on the outer layers; if your coconut oil feels thick and oily on your skin, change your brand.

On tropical islands coconut oil has been used as a skin moisturiser for thousands of years. For us, it is ideal for dry, rough and wrinkled skin. It prevents stretch marks and lightens existing ones. Its antiseptic elements keep the skin young and healthy and relatively free from infections. All of these benefits also make coconut oil ideal for massage and massage therapists.

As well as applying coconut oil to your skin, when you include it in your daily diet, through eating, drinking and using the many recipes offered in this book, you will benefit from its deep cleansing properties, its detox effects, balancing affects, and alkalising and antioxidant promoting factors – on the inside for your health, and on the outside for natural beauty.

Because of its MCFA content, coconut oil is incredibly versatile. Naturally anti-fungal, anti-microbial and anti-bacterial, coconut oil can be used as:

✔ A face cleanser

✔ An anti-bacterial alkaline toothpaste

✔ A deodorant

✔ A lip balm

✔ A cellulite treatment

✔ For cuticle and nail care.

Body synergy

If one part of your body isn't working at its best, this creates a chain reaction which then affects multiple systems in the body. If you have poor digestion, for example, not only will your body store fats and toxins in and around the organs, you're also limiting nutrient absorption in the body. It's surprising to think that some

overweight people are actually starving in their bodies, because no matter what they eat, their bodies cannot assimilate enough of the right nutrients. Their body holds onto fats because it's starving!

Over time, this damage becomes evident on the skin, hair and nails. You can tell a lot about a person's inner health by the look of their skin. For many years I experienced severe, chronic bouts of acne, mostly around my neck and chin. I later found out this was associated with digestive and hormonal problems.

Detoxification and the return of good digestive health results in natural weight loss, hormone balance, glowing skin and lustrous hair.

Moisturiser

The amount of oil used for face care will also vary for each individual. It's best to test this on your own skin. I know some women who swear by coconut oil as their only daily facial moisturiser. I personally find that three to four applications per week is enough. This might be because I have a Mediterranean constitution and my skin is quite naturally high in oils. I also eat a lot of coconut and other oils in my daily diet, which I am sure reduces my need for topical use.

Exfoliant

Coconut oil helps remove the layer of dead cells on the surface of your skin, making the skin look and feel smoother, lighter and more youthful. Mix it with some coarse sea salt to massage and gently exfoliate the skin.

Healthy hair

Polynesian, Asian and Pacific Island women often attribute their long, silky, shiny and rich-looking hair to the regular use of coconut oil as a hair conditioning treatment. Unlike many commercially-produced products, coconut oil offers moisture and hair nourishment that is both pure and nutrient-rich.

Coconut oil has a proven anti-microbial action and

contains small amounts of Vitamin E. This limits the amount of microorganisms in your scalp, which creates a healthy environment for hair growth (hence the long dark lustrous hair of Indian and Asian women).

Regular exposure to the elements and to the weather, and certain grooming techniques including brushing, shampooing, heat drying and colouring, can cause damage to the hair. Coconut oil can help reduce this kind of damage because of its ability to hydrate and lubricate the hair shaft. Due to its low molecular weight, coconut oil penetrates the hair cuticle, making it more effective than other hair oils which are heavier.

Coconut oil helps seal the moisture in hair, which reduces water loss and prevents dryness and breakage.

Hair is made of proteins – but that's just part of the story. At any given time, about 90% of your hair is in the growing phase – this can last anywhere from two to three years. At the end of that time, individual hairs enter a resting phase for about three months before they are shed and replaced by new ones. If you don't get enough protein in your diet, a disproportionate number of hairs may go into the resting phase, and increased hair shedding can occur two or three months later.

Coconut oil has been shown to reduce protein loss in hair, which is, of course, a huge benefit. Scientific studies have shown that protein loss is reduced when coconut oil is used as a moisturising pre-wash, rather than afterwards. Hair also retains its moisture better when treated in this way. Many oils may have the ability to lubricate hair, however only coconut oil has been shown to reduce hair damage due to protein loss.

Simply massage the coconut oil through your hair and leave it in as a treatment for two or more hours, then wash it out. You can also do this before bed and leave it in overnight. Each hair type will have different moisture requirements, so it is best that you determine for yourself how often your hair needs a treatment. I aim for at least one coconut oil hair treatment per week.

Natural beauty therapy

Try some of my natural, home-made beauty recipes made with Coconut Magic!

See the Coconut Body Care & Beauty recipes on page 228.

See Recipes for Coconut Oil Hair treatments in the Coconut Oil Body section page 229.

Chemical-free sunscreen

The light emitted by the sun consists of three frequency bands of radiation: infrared, visible and ultraviolet.

It is only the ultraviolet (UV) that can be harmful and cause sunburn.

There are two basic types of commercial sunscreen lotion on the market: products that penetrate the outermost layer of the skin to absorb UV rays, and products which coat the surface of the skin to act as physical barriers to UV rays. Both of these will be rated with a sun protection factor (SPF) number which lets you know how much protection is provided.

The chemical compounds that make up these SPF lotions are mostly synthetic and have a highly toxic effect on and in the body. Many commercial sunscreens may actually contribute to the development of cancer, because of their chemical additives. We are now coming back to grass roots and looking for healthier, natural remedies.

Foods to improve pH balance when eaten or applied topically include:

- ✓ Coconut oil – consume and apply topically

- ✓ Coconut vinegar – drink or apply topically

- ✓ Lemon – drink freshly-squeezed lemon

- ✓ Avocados – eat them to replenish good fats and natural liquids

- ✓ Leafy greens – a good dose of chlorophyll helps balance pH

- ✓ Coconut yoghurt – all yoghurts will be of benefit when eaten or applied topically

- ✓ Garlic – consume or apply topically for antibiotic properties.

So how does coconut oil offer skin protection? When applied topically its natural anti-microbial, anti-bacterial and anti-fungal properties will detoxify the outer layers of your skin. This will help to avoid the harmful chemical reaction these toxins can have when exposed to the sun's UV rays.

In his book *The Coconut Oil Miracle*, Dr Bruce Fife says, 'The first commercial suntan and sunscreen lotions contained coconut oil as their primary ingredient. Even today many sun screen lotions include coconut oil in their formulas. Coconut oil has an amazing ability to heal the skin and block the damaging effects of UV radiation from the sun. One of the reasons why it is so effective in protecting the skin is its antioxidant properties, which helps prevent burning and oxidative damage that promotes skin cancer.'

So why is it that it works wonders for some and not for others? The effectiveness of coconut oil in protecting you from sunburn depends also on your diet.

Dr Bruce Fife contends that when you eat large amounts of unsaturated oils they remain in your skin tissues, particularly polyunsaturated oils, as they are often hydrogenated and even rancid. Unsaturated oils are also heat- and light-sensitive (and therefore will oxidize easily). All these oils are highly vulnerable to peroxidation (the oxidative degradation of lipids) and contribute to sunburn. When an unsaturated oil is heated it becomes 'displaced' and is highly toxic in the body; this toxicity contributes to sunburn.

So to get the great effects of coconut oil as a natural sunscreen – keep your diet free from unhealthy fats and oils. Your skin can then remain clean and free from the micro-fungi and bacteria that these oils leave on your skin. Use coconut oil for cooking and consume coconut oil daily; this will help to detox your body, and prevent you from ingesting 'displaced oxidised oils'.

Warning: If you're not used to getting a lot of sun, it's a good idea to limit your exposure to start with, as your body needs to get used to producing its natural protective layers. Your body needs time to build up its natural tolerance.

COCONUT OIL AND SEX

There is another important use for coconut oil, and that's in the bedroom for sexual fun and health care.

Personal lubricant

A cooling tropical oil, coconut oil has an erotic aroma about it, and this can be just what you need to lift the mood for sexual intimacy. It can be used as a soothing and stimulating massage oil for both partners. It has many health benefits but most of all it can simply be used for fun.

Coconut oil also acts as a natural lubricant because it is very soothing to the skin, is a natural, non-toxic, light oil that has a mild, pleasant scent. Many commercial lubricants may contain parabens and other chemical ingredients – things that we know now to avoid, particularly on sensitive body parts!

Using coconut oil as a lubricant provides a safe, effective and natural moisture solution for those dry, intimate areas. The anti-bacterial, anti-viral, anti-fungal and anti-microbial benefits will also have health benefits. Although it does offer some protection for sexually transmitted diseases (STD), it is not recommended as an STD preventative.

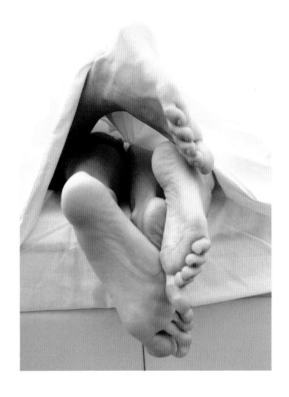

Warning

Coconut oil cannot be used in conjunction with latex condoms, as latex dissolves in coconut oil. Use polyurethane condoms instead. (If you use latex and rubber-based toys, also be careful!)

Vaginal health

Coconut oil is a great way to treat yeast infections as it contains caprylic acid, which has shown to be quite effective in combatting a variety of candida strains. Coconut oil can be applied directly to and inside the vagina since it is around the same pH level as a healthy vagina.

Coconut oil is safe internally, but make sure the coconut oil isn't spoiled; if it is, you could risk infection or make an existing infection worse. Spoiled coconut oil will look a bit like shattered glass, have cracks through it, and look a little fuzzy. Smell it! It should be pleasant and almost sweet. Check the bottom of the container for sediments or debris, which should not be there.

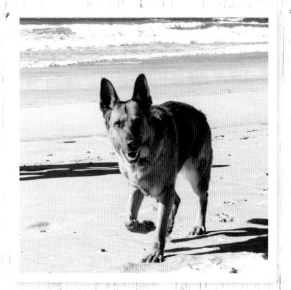

'Since adding coconut oil to our dog's diet it has helped Max immensely with his arthritis problems giving him more energy too. It is also good for his bad breath haha. It's true there are so many benefits for pets by adding coconut oil to their diet.'

Maria Kaye

'I use about 1-2 tablespoons in my dog's food to aid his digestion! Plus I put it on his fur to stop any dryness and brush it through to stop fleas.'

Rima Elmowy

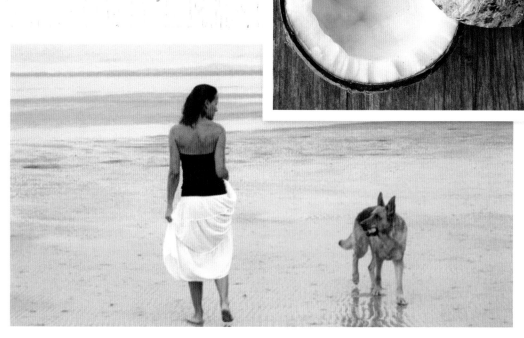

COCONUT OIL AND HEALTHY PETS

One morning at my local café I met a man and his dog. The German Shepherd looked quite sad; he was covered in skin lesions which were visible through his tatty fur. When I patted his head I could feel more skin disorders beneath his fur.

I chatted to the man and asked about his dog. He told me the dog was old – but it turned out he was only eight! He told me German Shepherds generally have skin disorders and I agreed, but mentioned that skin disorders are often a by-product of digestive disorders. I told him about my German Shepherd, Mocha, who is now approaching 12 years. She has immaculate skin and fur. Even though she is beginning to display signs of tiredness in her back legs, she continues to enjoy long beach walks and even plays with the ball every day.

He believed that the life span for a large dog was only around 10 years, but my dog is living proof that large dogs can live longer. I attribute her incredible health to Coconut Magic coconut oil in her daily diet, as well as raw food, including raw meats and vegetables, but no grains or processed foods. Her treats are all natural or fresh bones. Good sources of omega fatty acids, combined with coconut oil are also very effective for arthritis (in both humans and pets). The best way to feed a pet is to consider the type of diet they would have in the wild, because nature knows best. A diet in the wild does not include grains, tinned food or processed treats and dried food.

I've heard many success stories from owners feeding their pets coconut oil. And pets usually love it as I am sure that they intuitively know what's good for them.

For the past four years I have been feeding my dog coconut oil every day. Some days she eats it straight from my hand, other days I mix it in her evening meal.

Virtually every health benefit associated with coconut oil for humans is applicable also to animals.

Coconut oil can help your pet's digestion, improve their coat and build immune function, and has been shown to benefit all types of animals – dogs, cats, horses, cows and other farm animals.

Some of the benefits may include:

✔ Healthier skin and elimination of rashes

✔ Relief from arthritic symptoms

✔ Resolution of infections

✔ Healing of digestive issues

✔ Expulsion of worms

✔ Improved energy and vitality

✔ Healthy and shiny fur.

Applied topically, coconut oil helps with your pet's cuts, bites, stings and infections. Some people have even reported healing of serious ailments such as cancer and diabetes.

If your pet has never eaten coconut oil before, then start slowly, perhaps half a teaspoon for every 5 kg. If your pet is not used to eating fat it can cause loose stools; if everything is OK after a few days, gradually increase the dose to about one teaspoon per 5 kg. Puppies can start taking coconut oil in their food as soon as they start feeding. I feed Mocha (who is quite large) two tablespoons per day.

I am an animal lover, and super passionate about pet care. I cannot emphasise enough how beneficial it is to include coconut oil into your pet's diet. Also consider adding shredded coconut and fresh coconut meat, as they are both good sources of fibre.

WHAT THE EXPERTS ARE SAYING

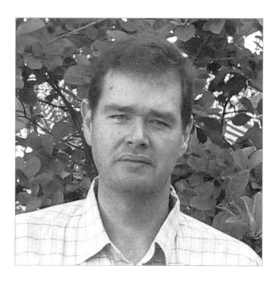

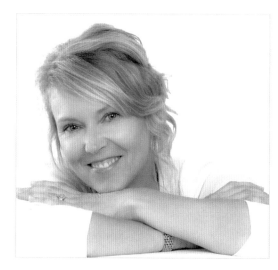

DAVID GILLESPIE

Author of *Toxic Oils*, *Big Fat Lies* and *Sweet Poison*. David is a 'recovering' corporate lawyer and co-founder of a software development company, as well as father to six young children. After trying every diet available, he found himself 40 kg overweight, and confused. So he set out to discover why he, like so many in his generation, was fat. He researched the truth about the food industry, labeling regulations and in particular in the industry of oils and sugars. What he discovered was that he had to stop poisoning himself. In his book *Toxic Oil* Gillespie exposes the myths in the health and diet industry, and presents a simple, safe answer to weight loss. David writes: 'To save you the bother of peering at label after label, I've taken a look at most of the cooking oils and fats you are likely to find on Australian supermarket shelves and listed the acceptable products based on their polyunsaturated fat content.' David listed Coconut Magic extra virgin coconut oil as the # No.1 cooking oil with only 0.1 g Polyunsaturated fat (grams per 100 ml).

www.davidgillespie.org

DELIA MCCABE

Author and keynote speaker, nutritional neuroscience researcher, specialist and leading authority on how nutrition, in particular fats and oils, affect brain cell function. Delia's 5 star review on Coconut Magic reads as follows: 'What great products – health, taste and integrity!! Coconut Magic produces the best coconut products that I have come across, because they understand the importance of keeping the fat molecules undamaged! The products are cold-pressed, organic, and the oil is stored in dark glass bottles. On top of this, their products are all sustainable, which means they are fostering Mother Earth, and causing no damage to the local environment where their coconuts are grown. I couldn't use any other coconut products! Thank you for going the extra mile with your business, and putting health at the top of your list of priorities.'

www.deliahealth.com

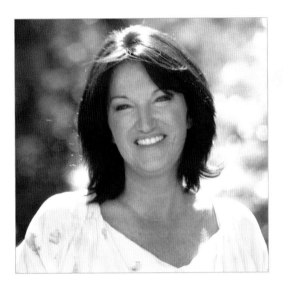

THERESE KERR

Best-selling author, a recognised holistic wellness advocate for Family Health, a visionary public speaker and health and well-being Ambassador for the Australian Certified Organic Organisation. Therese chooses Coconut Magic coconut oil in appreciation of its high quality and sustainable production technique. 'We love coconut oil, and Coconut Magic coconut oil is absolutely beautiful. I use it for my cooking and in my smoothies, a great addition to the health and well-being of any family and household.' Therese also enjoys the benefits of oil pulling therapy and loves to use coconut oil as a hair treatment. The Divine By Therese Kerr personal care products, and Divine Baby products use coconut oil as a key ingredient throughout their range.

www.theresekerr.com, www.thedivinecompany.com

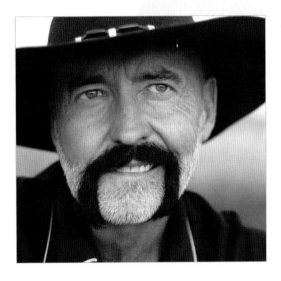

DON TOLMAN

Don Tolman has been referred to as a 'Modern Day Einstein' and is well known throughout international media as 'The Indiana Jones of Whole Foods'. Don is a renowned leader in the Wholefood Revolution and author of *The Farmacist Desk Reference I & II Encyclopedia of Wholefood Medicine*. Don Tolman and the team at Fortune Events choose Coconut Magic for its health promoting factors, superior quality, purity, taste and versatility. 'It is quite simply the best coconut oil available.'

www.dontolmaninternational.com and his Australian and New Zealand events at **www.fortuneevents.com**

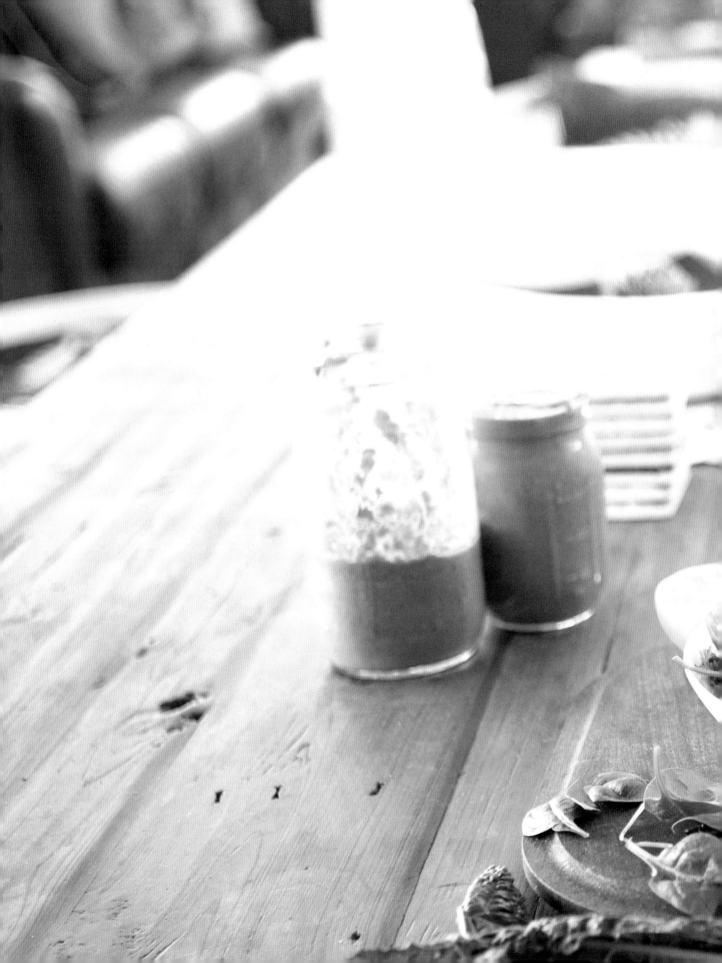

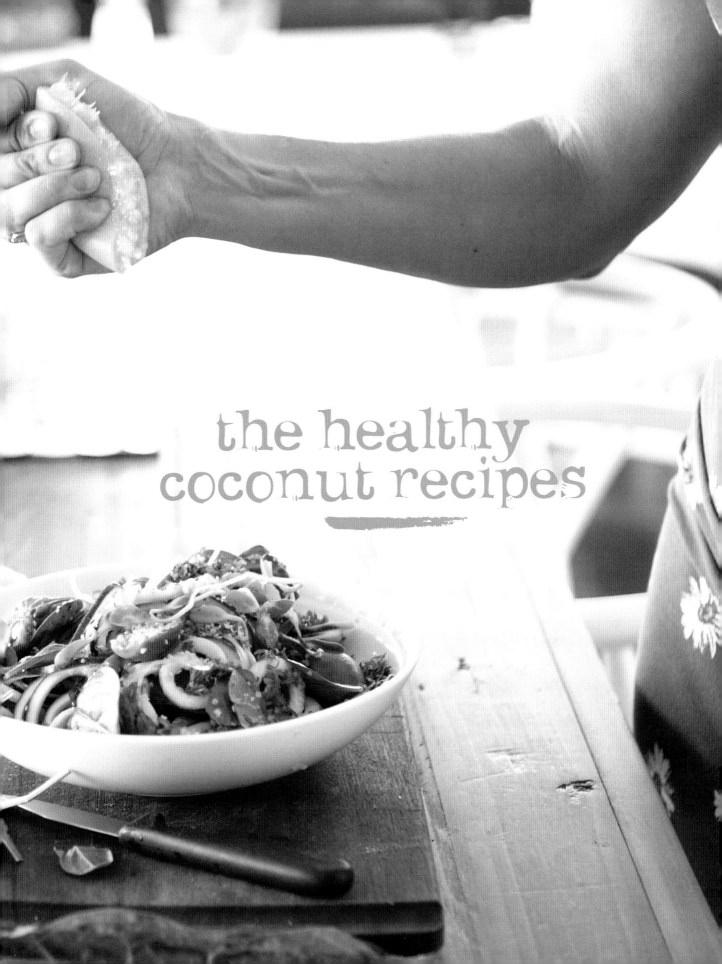

the healthy
coconut recipes

THE HEALTHY COCONUT RECIPES

The recipes featured in this book have been built around my own lifestyle/diet, which is predominantly centred on plant-based foods. I created many of the recipes in this book over several years, as I experimented with coconut products and other healthy ingredients. The team at Coconut Magic has also contributed, and our food blogger friends and communities inspire me daily with their coconutty creations and beautiful food images.

I have also included a selection of raw foods, because for 30 days every year my husband and I focus on eating only delicious, raw meals. I have included some of the recipes that I learned while living in Thailand, and from my involvement with the local raw food workshops at Spa Samui.

The work of nutritionists and health ambassadors, David Wolfe, Gabrielle Cousens, Brendan Brazier, Don Tolman and Tyler Tolman have contributed enormously to my education; they have inspired me in my desire to live a plant-based, high-nutrition lifestyle. I have also had the pleasure of working closely with Don and Tyler Tolman, and Fortune Events in spreading the coconut love.

Plant Based Nutrition

There is a lot of conflicting and confusing information out there: eat dairy, don't eat dairy. Eat meat, don't eat meat. Eat soy, don't eat soy...and on it goes.

Thankfully, in all my years of research, I have found one common thread. All health educators agree that a diet high in plant-based nutrition is beneficial to our health. And so the recipes in this book are designed to help you achieve that for yourself and for your family.

Although not all recipes include coconut or coconut oil, most do. The overall theme of the recipes are:

- ✓ High in nutritional plant-based food content

- ✓ Plenty of healthy oils

- ✓ No refined or processed foods

- ✓ Using coconut sweeteners as a natural sugar alternative

- ✓ All are vegan, gluten, wheat, dairy and soy free.

Clean Water

Many recipes refer to 'clean water' – this can be spring water or a good source of filtered water, in which fluoride and chlorine are both removed.

'The most important ingredient to add to any dish is love.'

Pink Salt

I prefer to use pink salt in my recipes, because these salts are unrefined and still retain some of their mineral content.

Melting your Coconut Oil

Many recipes will require melted coconut oil. To do this, simply place your jar of oil into a saucepan of warm to hot water. If your oil comes in a plastic container, transfer to a glass jar to melt. Do not microwave your coconut oil as this will damage vital nutrients.

Activating Nuts

Raw nuts are a fantastic healthy snack, loaded with protein, healthy fats, fibre and important minerals like zinc, magnesium and calcium. However, nuts also contain natural chemicals that can interfere with the absorption of these nutrients. Raw nuts contain phytic acid and enzyme inhibitors that can reduce the body's ability to absorb certain nutrients properly.

Eating large amounts of raw nuts can put extra pressure on your digestive system and may cause uncomfortable digestive symptoms like bloating, heaviness and nausea. The best way to resolve these issues is to activate your nuts. Simply soaking them for a few hours, then giving them a good wash with clean water is enough to remove the digestive inhibitor chemicals.

Soaking and Sprouting Grains and Legumes

Soaking neutralises the enzyme inhibitors present in dry grains, seeds and legumes, and starts the production of numerous beneficial enzymes. As they soak, the enzymes, lactobacilli and other helpful organisms break down and neutralise the phytic acid. As little as seven hours soaking in water removes most of the phytic acid.

To sprout a grain, seed or bean, first wash then soak in cool to tepid filtered or spring water. Soaking time varies between 4 and 12 hours, depending on the size and hardness of the seed. Large, hard beans such as garbanzo beans need 12 hours, whereas small, soft seeds like lentils, buckwheat, amaranth, quinoa and many vegetable seeds only need four hours. Rinse and change the water every couple of hours while they soak.

Drain and keep them moist. I put mine in a closed container in the fridge and rinse them a couple of times each day. You can also put them in a jar covered with cheesecloth and secured with a rubber band. The seeds need to be kept damp and aired, but not wet, otherwise there is a chance of mould or spoiling.

Some seeds start to sprout in a few hours. Within two to five days most of the bigger seeds, nuts and beans are ready. (You can tell they are ready when the root – not the shoot, which is longer – is the length of the seed.) Keep your sprouting seeds and grains out of full sunlight. Natural light is OK, but full sunlight will encourage leaves to grow.

It is best to use only organic produce when sprouting. Non-organic produce is made with chemicals and they may not sprout.

smoothies, juices & teas

smoothies

Adding Coconut Oil to Your Smoothies

When you add a tablespoon of coconut oil to your smoothie, you increase the nutritional content and you include a great source of fat. If you make your smoothies with fruit (which contain fructose), coconut oil will stop your blood sugars from spiking. Coconut oil helps your body to absorb vital and fat-soluble nutrients.

Preparing Your Smoothie

Smoothies are a great addition to your healthy lifestyle. A smoothie delivers a blast of wholefood and superfood nutrition, with all phytonutrients broken down so that your body can readily absorb them.

Greens are important! Most of us don't get enough dark green leafy vegetables in our daily diet, but it is important to alternate your greens regularly.

The basis for a great green smoothie includes:

2 cups dark leafy greens: alternate kale, spinach, lettuce, silver beet, collards, bok choy

2 cups liquid: water, coconut water, almond milk, coconut milk

3 cups fresh fruits: banana, mango, berries, grapefruit, orange, avocado, peach, pear, pineapple, apple, lemons and lime

Adding superfood boosters increases nutrient intake.

These include: Coconut oil, goji, acai berry powder, macqui berry powder, maca powder, chia seeds, nuts, hemp seeds, cinnamon, flax, and cacao powder

Blend the greens and liquid together, then add the superfoods and fruits to the mix. Add the coconut oil whilst blending and use either ice or some frozen fruit to chill the smoothie.

coconut chai spice

choc mint blast

coconut belly soother

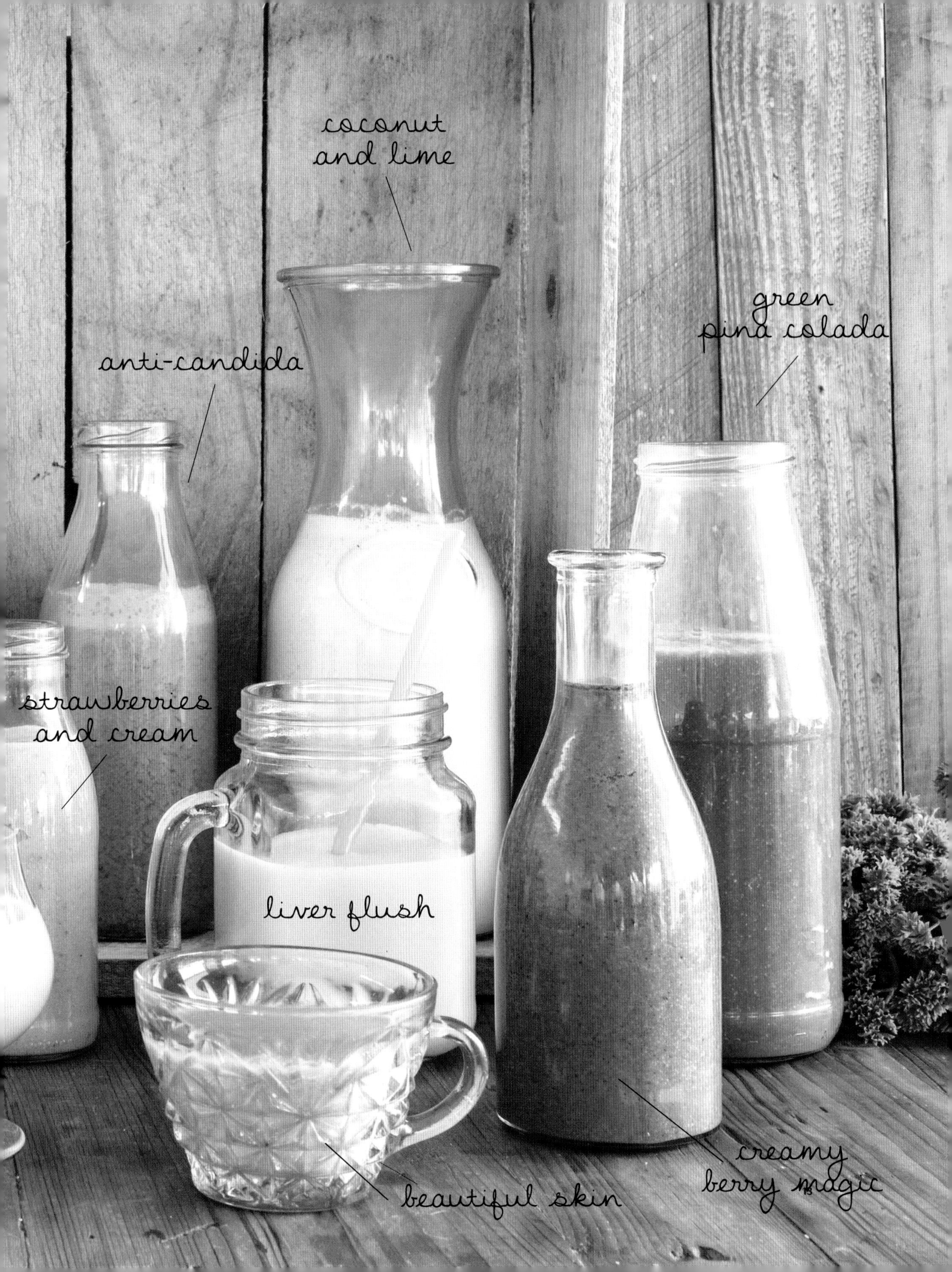

coconut
and lime

green
pina colada

anti-candida

strawberries
and cream

liver flush

creamy
berry magic

beautiful skin

coconut smoothies

CHAI SPICE

½ cup cashews

2 cups coconut water

2 dates, pitted

2 tbs Coconut Magic coconut oil

2 tbs Coconut Magic desiccated coconut

2 tbs maca powder

1 tsp cinnamon powder

1 tsp ginger powder

½ tsp cardamom powder or 2 drops
of cardamom liquid

1 large frozen banana or 2 cups frozen coconut meat

1 cup of ice

Blend all ingredients together except for the frozen banana/coconut meat and ice. Add the frozen items once all other items are blended.

Serves 2 medium cups

ANTI - CANDIDA DRINK

1 small clove of garlic

1 tbs Coconut Magic coconut oil

1 handful of dark leafy greens

1 cup clean water

Juice of one lemon

Blend all ingredients except lemon. When smooth, add lemon juice and mix well.

Serves 1 glass

GREEN PINA COLADA

2 cups dark green spinach leaves

1 cup pineapple, chopped into small pieces

1 banana

5-6 fresh mint leaves

1½ cups of ice

2 tbs Coconut Magic desiccated coconut

½ cup clean water

2 tbs Coconut Magic coconut oil

Blend all ingredients except for the coconut oil for one minute, starting slowly and building up speed. After a minute, add the coconut oil whilst continuing to blend. Add clean water if required to your desired consistency.

Serves 2 cups

COCONUT BELLY SOOTHER

1 cup papaya

1 cup coconut water

¼ cup coconut yoghurt

1 small lime, peeled

1 tbs Coconut Magic coconut nectar
(optional to sweeten as desired)

2 tbs Coconut Magic coconut oil

Blend all ingredients except the coconut oil in a high speed blender. After a minute or two, add the coconut oil and blend until smooth.

Makes 2 small serves

LIVER FLUSH

If a flatter belly is on your wish list, start with this ultra-cleansing and digestive support drink. I came across this recipe whilst detoxing at the Spa Samui retreat in Thailand. Ginger and garlic have very good natural anti-viral and anti-inflammatory properties to help build your immune system. This drink tastes surprisingly good and refreshing.

1 cup fresh orange juice

1 tbs lime juice

1 clove garlic

1 slice ginger

1 tbs olive oil

1 tbs Coconut Magic coconut oil

1 pinch (1/5 tsp) Cayenne pepper

Blend all ingredients in a high speed blender for about 1 minute. If you like more of a bite, you can add more garlic and ginger.

Serves 1 glass

COCONUT AND LIME

1 cup coconut milk

1 cup ice

¼ cup cashews

3 limes, juice only

1 banana

2 tsp Coconut Magic desiccated coconut

2 tbs Coconut Magic coconut oil

1-2 Medjool dates

Blend all ingredients except the coconut oil in a high speed blender, starting slowly and building up speed. After a minute or two, add the coconut oil and blend. Add the ice and water and blend until smooth.

Serves 2 glasses

BEAUTIFUL SKIN

This is a gluten-free, golden ticket to a clear complexion! Coconut water restores radiance with live electrolytes. Parsley oxygenates, cucumber revitalises, coconut oil moisturises, lemon provides toning vitamin C, and mint packs vitamin A, which strengthens skin tissue and helps reduce oily skin. Hemp seeds are a balanced source of omega rich fatty acids.

1 cucumber, peeled and chopped

1 pear, chopped

1 green apple, chopped

2 cups clean water or coconut water

1 cup dark green spinach leaves

1 cup romaine lettuce

2 tbs hemp seeds

1 banana

2 tbs parsley

3-4 fresh mint leaves

2 tbs Coconut Magic coconut oil

1 lemon, juice only

Place apple, pear and cucumber into a bowl and set aside. Add green leaves, hemp seeds and water to the blender, start blending at a low speed. Add pear, apple and cucumber and blend again. Add banana, parsley, mint leaves, coconut oil and continue to blend until all ingredients are well combined. Finally add the squeezed lemon juice and serve.

Serves 2 glasses

CREAMY BERRY MAGIC

1 cup blueberries

2 tbs cacao powder

½ avocado

1 tsp vanilla essence

1½ cups coconut milk

½ cup ice

2 tbs Coconut Magic coconut nectar

(or as sweet as you like it)

2 tbs Coconut Magic coconut oil

Blend all ingredients except for the coconut oil for one minute, starting slowly and building up speed. After a minute, add the coconut oil whilst continuing to blend. Add clean water if required to your desired consistency. Add cacao nibs and coconut flakes to garnish.

Serves 2 glasses

CHOC MINT BLAST

2 cups cold almond milk

2 tbs cacao powder

6 fresh mint leaves

1 large banana, frozen

1-2 tbs Coconut Magic coconut nectar

1 tbs cacao nibs

½ cup cashews for a thicker consistency

2 tbs Coconut Magic coconut oil

Optional: 1 tbs matcha green tea powder

Blend all ingredients except the coconut oil in a high speed blender. After a minute or two, add the coconut oil and blend until smooth.

Serves 2 glasses

STRAWBERRIES AND CREAM

A delicious superfood blend!

1 cup fresh organic strawberries

1 cup coconut water

¾ cup raw cashews

1 large frozen banana

2 tbs Coconut Magic coconut oil

1 pinch nutmeg

1 pinch cinnamon

Blend all ingredients except for the coconut oil for one minute, starting slowly and building up speed. After a minute, add the coconut oil whilst continuing to blend. Add clean water if required to your desired consistency.

Add cacao nibs and coconut flakes to garnish.

Serves 2 glasses

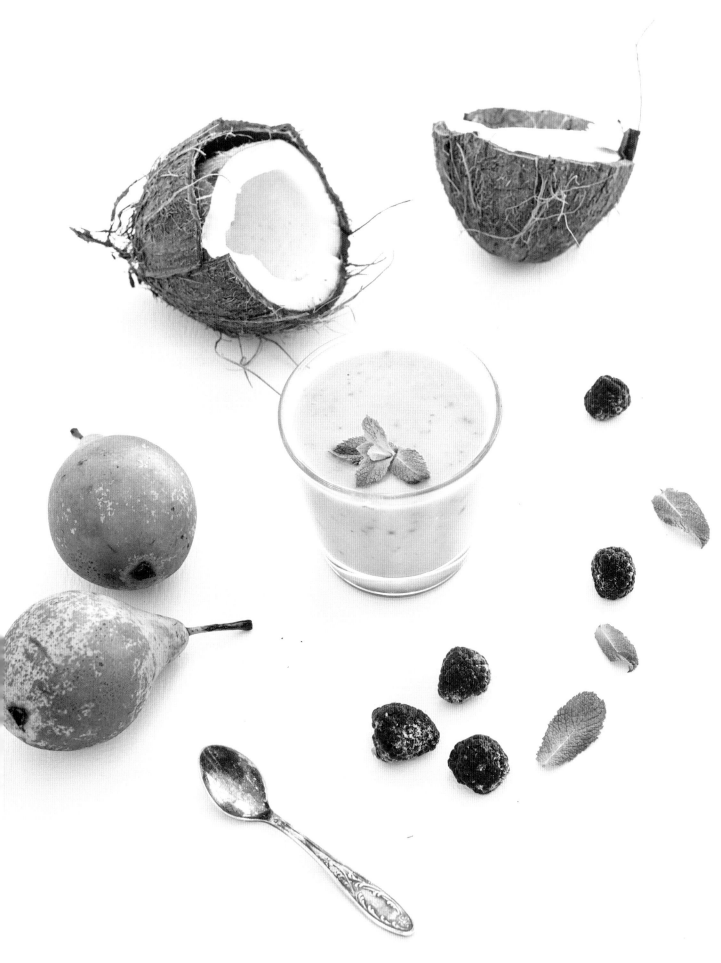

coconut teas

Tea is soothing and warming. Herbs, spices and even coconut oil can be added to your tea recipes making tea an incredibly healthy drink.

GINGER COCONUT TEA

Fresh ginger, sliced finely

1 tbs Coconut Magic coconut oil

Coconut Magic coconut sugar
to sweeten (optional)

Place ginger and sugar in cup. Slowly add boiling water. Add coconut oil and stir well.

Serves 2 glasses

COCONUT LEMON DETOX

Drink as a morning detox or as a cleansing and energising drink any time of the day.

Juice of ½ lemon

1 tbs Coconut Magic coconut oil

1 cup of clean water

Into a mug, add about 2 tbs room-temperature water. (This is so you don't blast the lemon with hot water.) Add coconut oil and lemon juice.

Add hot water, stirring as you do. As you stir, the coconut oil will blend.

Serves 1 glass

GREEN MINT TEA

2 slices of lemon

4 mint leaves

2 tbs Coconut Magic coconut oil

2 tbs organic green tea leaves

2 cups clean water

Add green tea leaves and water to a small pot on medium heat and slowly bring to a boil.

Take off the heat and add remaining ingredients. Stir well and serve.

Serves 2 glasses

COCONUT MAGIC LATTE

1 tbs dandelion root, roasted

¾ cup boiled water

2 tbs Coconut Magic coconut oil

1 tsp Coconut Magic coconut sugar or nectar (optional to taste)

½ tsp vanilla essence (optional)

Using a coffee plunger, brew the dandelion in the hot water for 2-3 minutes.

Once brewed, add all ingredients to the blender, and blend for 30 seconds or until the mixture becomes creamy and frothy. Serve immediately.

Serves: adjust as required

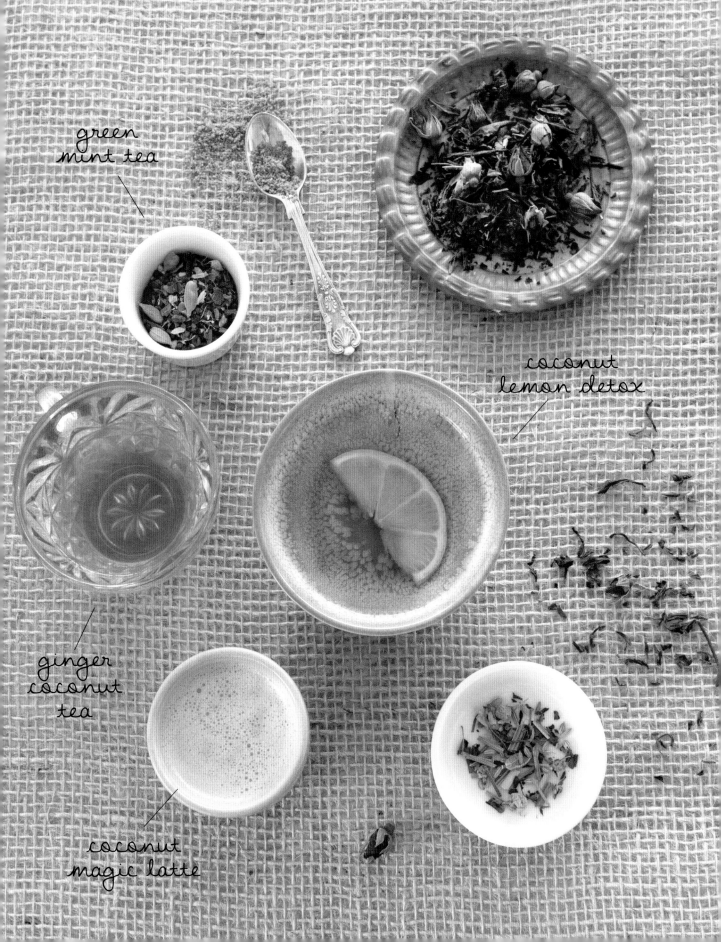

green
mint tea

coconut
lemon detox

ginger
coconut
tea

coconut
magic latte

juicing for health

Juicing offers a blast of nutrition, including essential vitamins and minerals, which can assist in healing the body, especially when taken on an empty stomach. It's almost like an intravenous vitamin injection!

These easy juicing recipes are a great way to lose weight and have more energy. They're tailored to be pleasing to the palate, yet still providing you with the important nutrients from dark leafy greens.

WAKE ME UP GREEN JUICE

Add a zing of ginger to your morning routine! This is a healthy, cleansing and energising drink. Cucumber is full of silica, which energises the immune system and is great for hair, skin and nails. Buy organic when you can, and keep the skin on.

1 bunch kale

1 whole cucumber

2 green apples

1 lemon, peeled

1 slice ginger

Handful of mint or parsley

Wash ingredients well. If organic, retain the skin on the cucumber. If commercially grown, peel.

Juice all ingredients.

Stir and drink as soon as possible.

NB: You can substitute the kale for 5-6 celery stalks - I like to juice these with the celery leaves.

Serves 2 glasses

BODY BEET

I drink one of these almost every day. This is a must for a daily alkaline balance.

1 beetroot, washed and peeled

2 apples

3 carrots

1 lemon, peeled

Wash ingredients well and juice.

Serves 1-2 glasses

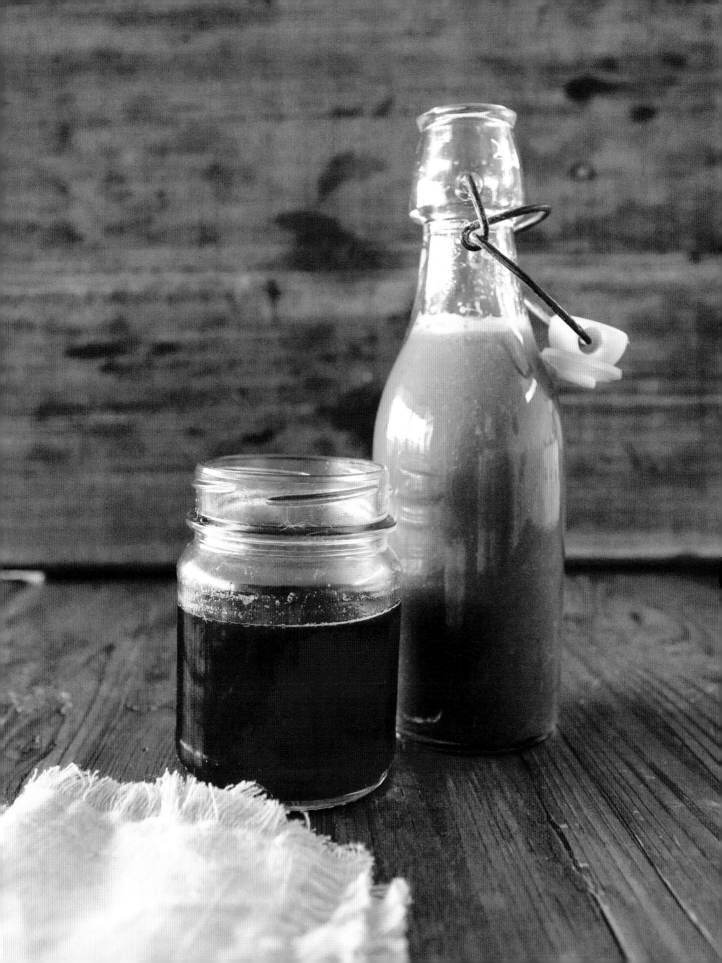

breakfast

FLUFFY COCONUT FLOUR PANCAKES

Coconut is a good source of energy and therefore a great way to start your first meal of the day.

4 chia eggs (4 tbs chia seeds
and 1 cup of clean water)

2 cups coconut milk or almond milk

2 tsp vanilla extract

1 tbs Coconut Magic coconut nectar

½ cup almond meal or buckwheat flour

½ cup Coconut Magic coconut flour

¼ cup arrowroot powder

1 tsp cinnamon powder

½ tsp pink salt

1 tsp baking powder

2 tbs Coconut Magic desiccated coconut

¼ cup clean water

3-4 tbs Coconut Magic coconut oil
for frying

Wet Ingredients:

Prepare the chia eggs by placing the chia seeds in a bowl with one cup of water. Set aside for 15 minutes so that it forms a gel.

Once the chia gel is ready mix in coconut (or almond) milk, vanilla extract and coconut nectar.

Dry Ingredients:

Sift the coconut flour, buckwheat flour (or almond meal) , arrowroot, cinnamon, salt and baking powder into a medium-sized bowl. Stir in the desiccated coconut.

Add the wet mixture to the dry mixture until the coconut flour is completely incorporated.

Grease pan with coconut oil. Using a few tablespoons of the batter prepare into pancake shapes and place into pan. The pancakes should be 2-3 inches in diameter and fairly thick. (Keep the pancakes small for a fluffier result.)

Cook for a few minutes on each side, until the tops dry out slightly and the bottoms start to brown. Flip and cook an additional 2-3 minutes.

Makes 10 small fluffy pancakes + prep: 15 min. setting: 10 min.

Optional

Slice some fresh banana on top of your pancakes and serve with a drizzle of Coconut Magic coconut nectar.

Acai Berry Coconut Ice Cream is also a lovely side serve for the pancakes (see page 214, for the recipe). The pancake mix will store in the fridge for up to three days. Once cooked, pancakes should be served immediately.

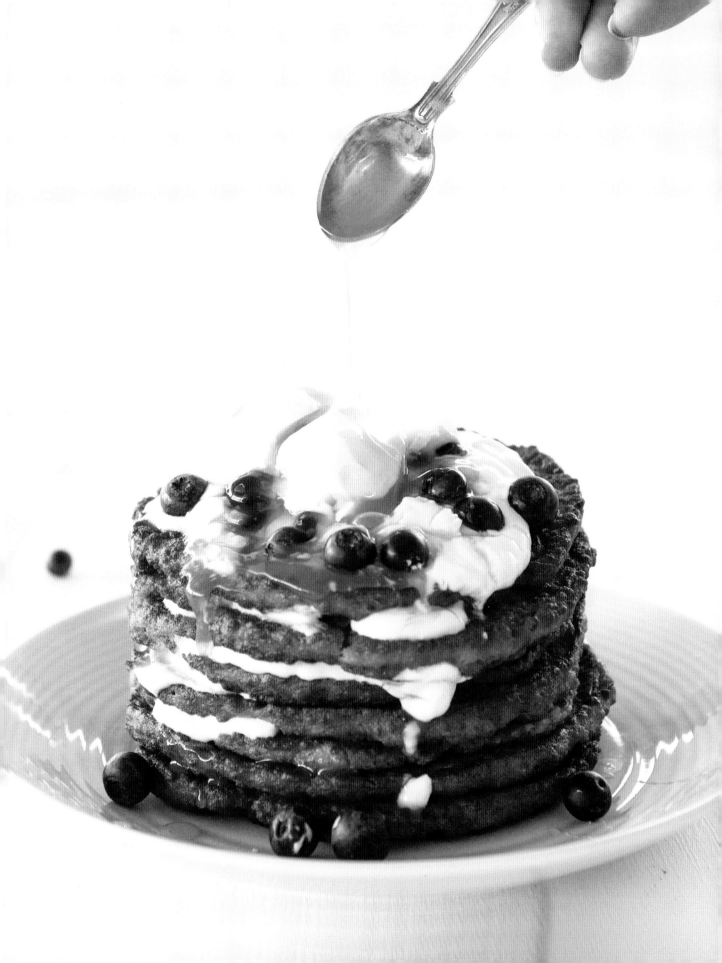

COCONUT OIL BREAKFAST BARS

½ cup almond butter

½ cup coconut butter

½ cup Coconut Magic coconut nectar

½ cup Coconut Magic coconut oil

2½ cups quinoa flakes

1 cup Coconut Magic coconut flakes

¼ cup dried mulberries (optional)
– any dried fruit, nuts or seeds

¼ cup goji berries (optional)
– any dried fruit, nuts or seeds

¼ cup cacao nibs (optional)

In a medium pot set over medium-low heat, melt together almond butter, coconut butter, coconut nectar and coconut oil, stirring until smooth.

Remove from stove and stir in quinoa flakes and shredded coconut. Add dried fruit, cacao nibs, nuts or seeds – your choice!

Pour mixture into a 9- by 13-inch baking dish. Spread into an even layer, sprinkle with mini cacao nibs (if using), and firmly press down with the back of a spatula or clean hands.

Refrigerate for 2 hours or until firm.

Slice into squares or bars, 3 rows of 4 bars each, and remove from the pan.

Store breakfast bars in the refrigerator, either in an airtight container with wax paper separating the layers, or individually wrapped in plastic wrap. They will keep for 7-10 days.

Makes 12 bars + prep: 30 min. + setting time: 2 hours

Optional

You may add chopped nuts, seeds, and/or dried fruit. You can even add some raw chocolate to the mixture allowing it to completely melt, to make Chocolate and Coconut Breakfast Bars.

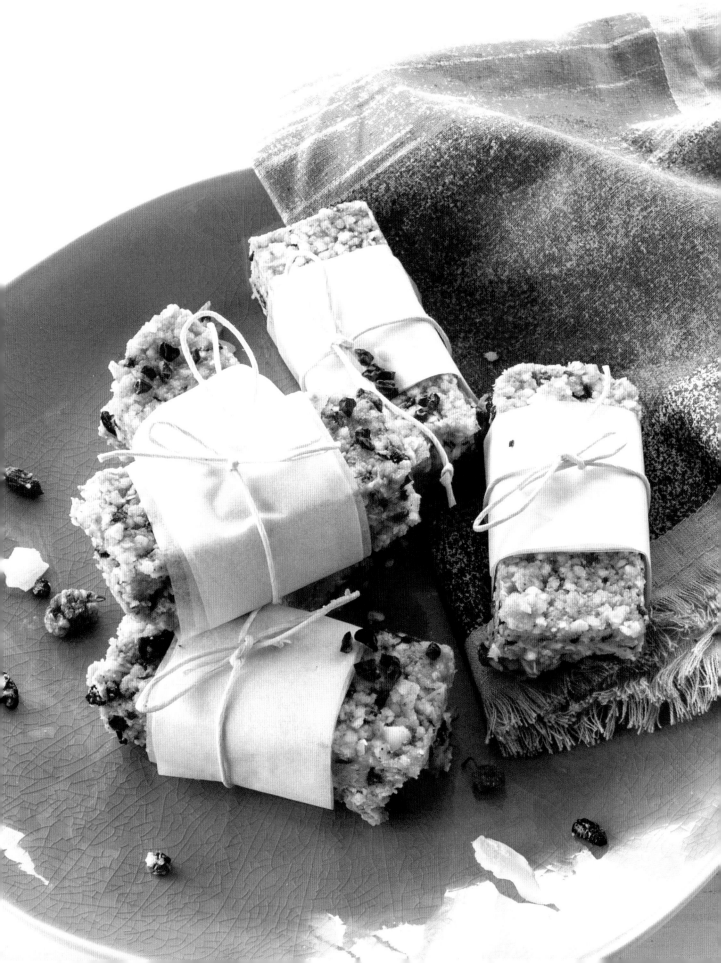

COCONUT CEREAL

This easy homemade Coconut Cereal is great with coconut yoghurt or by the handful!

2 cups quinoa flakes

¾ cup Coconut Magic coconut flakes

½ cup chopped almonds

⅓ cup pepitas

2 tbs Coconut Magic coconut sugar

1 tsp cinnamon

¼ tsp pink salt

1 tsp vanilla extract

4 tbs Coconut Magic coconut oil, melted

½ cup Coconut Magic coconut nectar

¼ cup clean water

Preheat the oven to 150°C (300°F).

Line a large baking tray with parchment paper. Set aside.

In a medium-sized bowl mix all the dry ingredients – everything except the coconut oil, coconut nectar and water. Stir together until well combined.

In a small bowl mix together the melted coconut oil, coconut nectar and water.

Add the wet ingredients to the dry ingredients.

Mix well and then spread over the baking sheet.

Bake the cereal in the oven for about 30-40 minutes, or until it becomes golden brown and crunchy, stirring half way through.

Let the cereal cool on the baking sheet.

Serve with fresh fruit such as diced apple or mango, and nut milk or coconut yoghurt.

Store in an airtight container for up to 1 month.

Makes 8-10 breakfast servings, or about 5 cups granola
+ prep: 10 min. + cooking: 60 min. + cooling: 30 min.

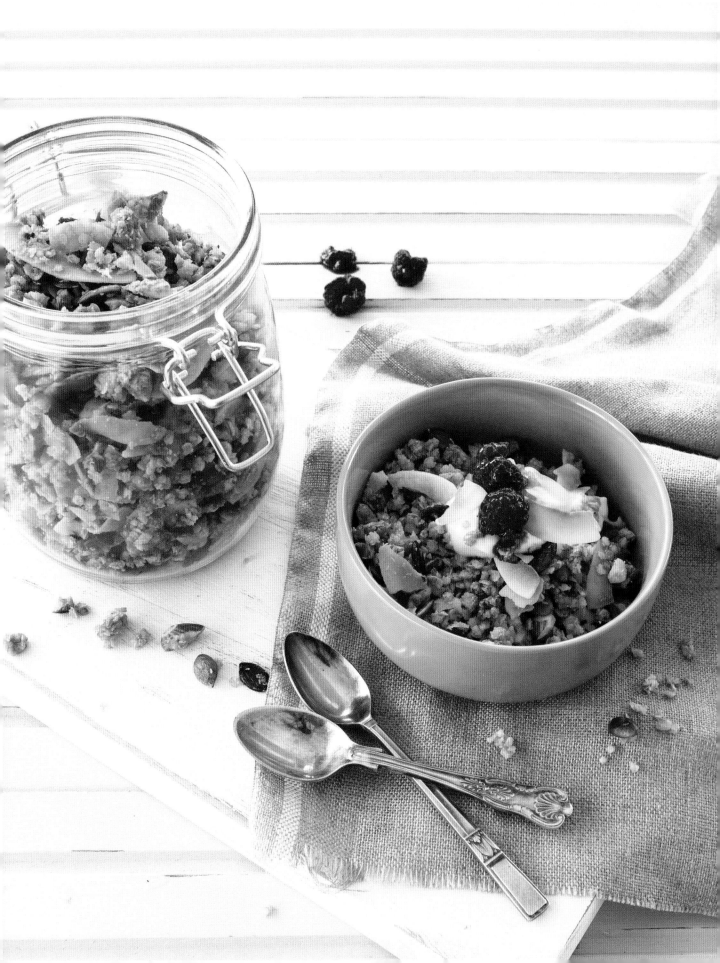

CINNAMON & COCONUT QUINOA PORRIDGE WITH WALNUT AND CURRANTS

Coconut quinoa porridge can be eaten after a meal as a dessert or as a sweet and warming breakfast. Add some sliced banana and other fresh fruit or nuts of your choice to garnish.

1 cup quinoa

1½ cups coconut milk

½ cup clean water

2 tsp ground cinnamon

2 tbs Coconut Magic coconut nectar (to your taste)

¼ cup currants or raisins

2 tbs Coconut Magic coconut oil

¼ cup walnuts, chopped into small pieces

Wash the quinoa and rinse well.

In a medium saucepan, over a medium heat, combine the coconut milk and water and bring to the boil.

Add the quinoa, cover and simmer for 10 minutes. The water will begin to be absorbed by the quinoa.

Add the cinnamon and coconut nectar and continue to simmer for another 5 minutes or until all of the water is completely absorbed.

Remove from the heat and mix through the currants (or raisins), coconut oil and walnuts.

Serves: 2 large or 4 small bowls + prep: 20 min. + cooking: 15 min.

Optional

Add some raw cacao powder for a chocolate flavoured porridge.

Serve with fresh fruit – bananas or fresh berries will work well.

Garnish with 1 tbs Coconut Magic coconut flakes for an added crunch.

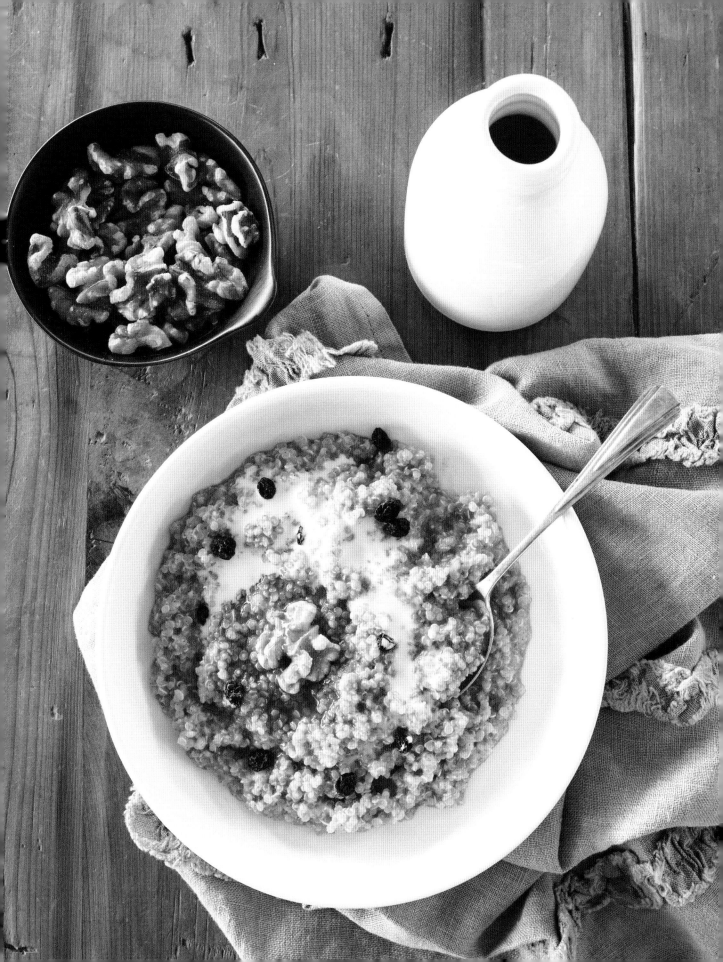

CHOC CHIA & HEMP BOWL

PUDDING

½ cup hemp seeds

1 cup coconut milk

2 tbs Coconut Magic coconut nectar

2 tbs Coconut Magic coconut oil, melted

¼ cup cacao powder

1 tsp pure vanilla extract

¼ tsp pink salt

½ cup chia seeds

TOPPINGS

½ cup fresh raspberries

Pinch of vanilla seeds (optional)

Pinch of sesame seeds (optional)

1 tbs coconut yoghurt per serve (store bought or see page 112 for the recipe)

Pistachio nuts, cacao nibs and berries to garnish

Blend all of the pudding ingredients in the blender, except for the chia seeds, until creamy and smooth.

Put the liquid from the blender into a container. Add the chia seeds.

Place in the fridge for 1-2 hours.

The pudding will set as the chia seeds expand. Serve with your choice of topping.

serves 2 + prep: 10 min. + setting time: 1-2 hrs

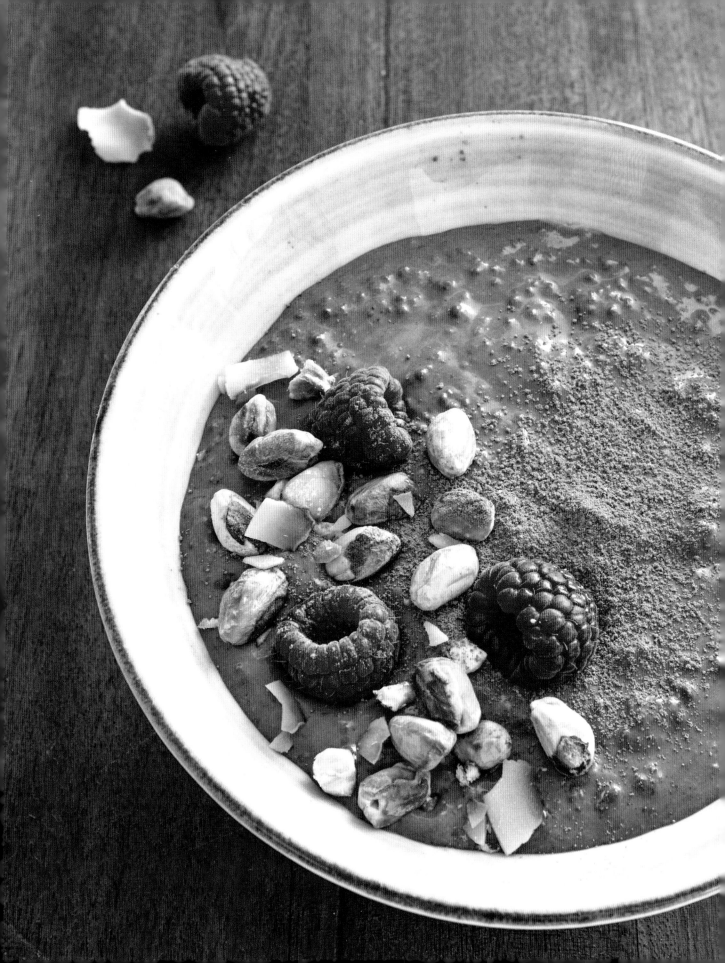

BERRY & PEAR CRUMBLE WITH VANILLA CASHEW CREAM

VANILLA CASHEW CREAM

1 cup raw cashews, soaked for 1-2 hours

¼ cup pecan nuts

¼ cup Coconut Magic coconut nectar

¼ cup Coconut Magic coconut oil

¼ tsp vanilla paste

½ cup clean water

BERRIES

250g punnet strawberries,
washed then halved or quartered

125g punnet blueberries, washed

1 pear, thinly sliced

CRUMBLE

¼ cup raw almonds

¼ cup raw cashews

¼ cup Coconut Magic coconut flakes

¼ cup quinoa flakes

1 tbs Coconut Magic coconut nectar

¼ tsp ground cinnamon

Vanilla Cashew Cream:

Wash and rinse the soaked cashews. Place all ingredients in a blender or use a sticker mixer and blend on high for 4 minutes, or until smooth. Refrigerate and set aside.

Crumble:

Place the almonds and cashews in a small food processor and process until finely chopped.

Transfer to a bowl and add the remaining ingredients.

To serve, divide the fruit between four bowls.

Spoon over the cashew cream and crumble mixture.

Drizzle with extra Coconut Magic coconut nectar.

Serves 2 large or 4 small bowls + prep: 15 min.

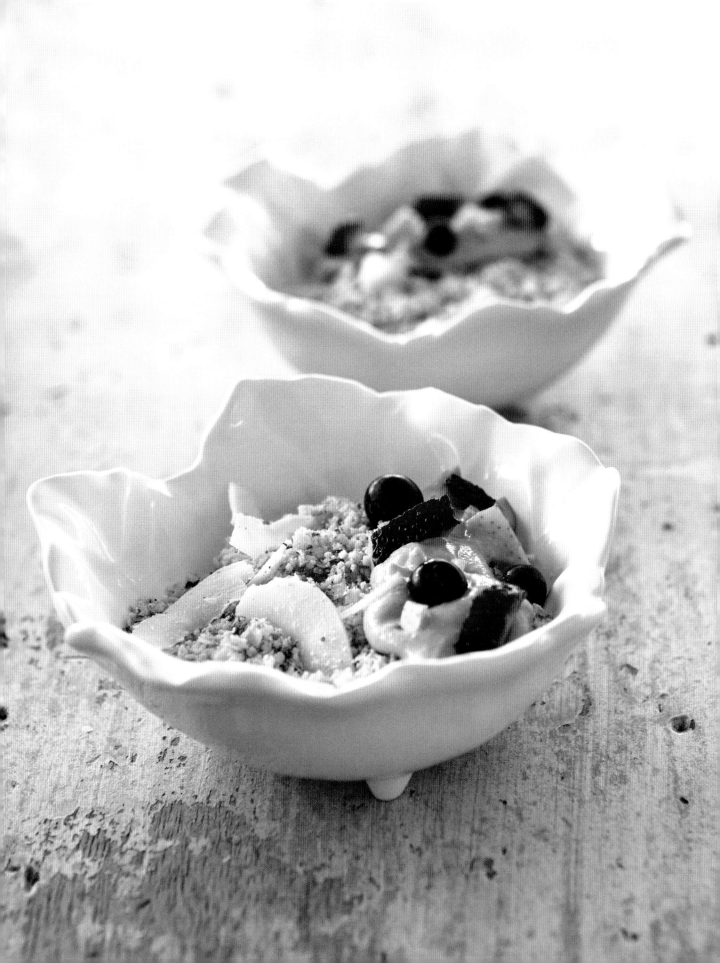

BUCKWHEAT WRAPS

I first tried these delicious gluten-free wraps when visiting Kamalaya Resort, a very special Wellness Sanctuary and Holistic Spa in Koh Samui, Thailand. The recipe is by The Healthy Chef, Teresa Cutter. Teresa assisted the spa with the development of their recipes and detox programs. If you like this recipe you can see more from Teresa Cutter at www.thehealthychef.com

Buckwheat is gluten-free as well as high in protein and essential minerals. The juice is high in nutrition and with just a few basic ingredients these wraps are very easy to make.

300 ml carrot juice

1 cup buckwheat flour

1 tbs arrowroot powder

Pinch nutmeg

Pinch pink salt

Coconut Magic coconut oil for frying

Pour juice into a bowl. Whisk in the buckwheat flour until combined.

Whisk in the arrowroot and season with the nutmeg and sea salt. Check the consistency – it should flow like a crepe batter. You can adjust by adding a little more buckwheat flour or juice if necessary.

Lightly oil a pan with a little coconut oil, then pour just enough batter to coat the bottom of the pan. Cook for 1 minute and flip over with a spatula. Cook the other side for a few more seconds.

Cool the wraps on a plate and store between sheets of grease-proof paper.

Store wrapped in the fridge for up to 3 days.

Makes 5 wraps + prep: 25 min. cook: 3-5 min.

Optional

Use green juice for a lovely green coloured wrap (kale and zucchini works well).

Add fresh chopped garden herbs or a little cayenne pepper to the wrap mix before cooking to boost flavor.

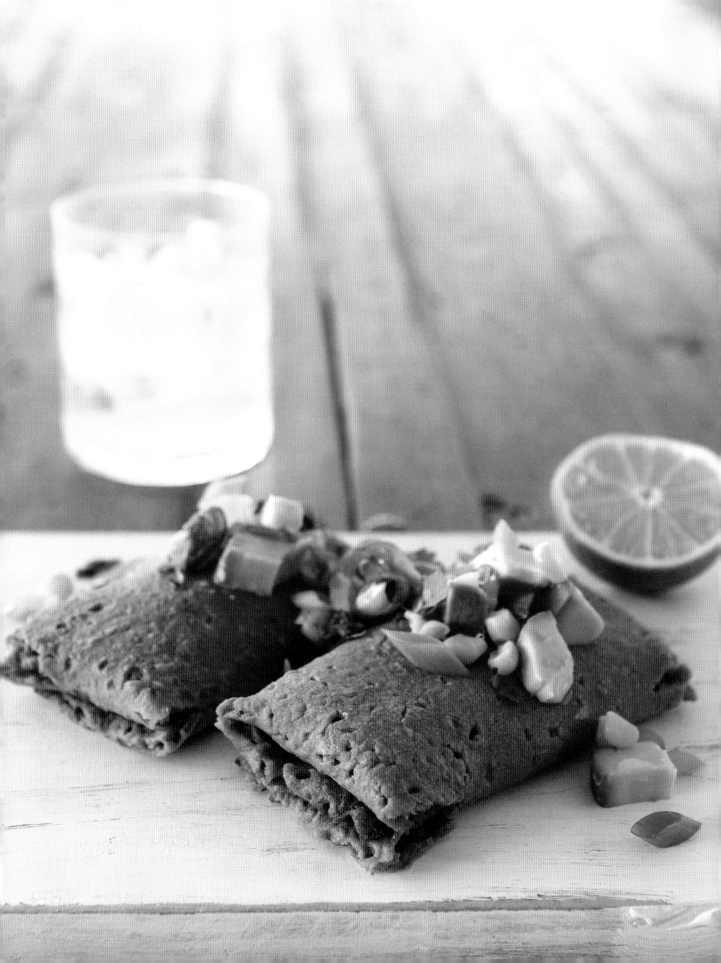

COCONUT BREAD WITH CHIA JAM

Coconut bread can be eaten with any of your favourite toppings, including coconut oil! It's nice to have with a warm herbal tea, fresh juice, or a berry smoothie. Serve with chia jam and/or a drizzle of coconut nectar.

3 tbs chia seeds soaked in 1 cup of water to make chia gel

1 cup Coconut Magic coconut flour

½ cup Coconut Magic coconut oil

½ cup buckwheat flour

1 pinch of pink salt

¼ cup walnuts, finely chopped

½ tsp cinnamon powder

1 tbs Coconut Magic coconut nectar

2 tbs Coconut Magic coconut sugar

1 tsp baking powder (aluminium free)

¼ cup Coconut Magic desiccated coconut

BERRY CHIA JAM

1 cup of organic berries, washed

2 tbs clean water

2 tbs Coconut Magic coconut nectar

2 tbs chia seeds

½ lemon, juiced

Coconut Bread:

Using a medium sized bowl add the chia seeds to the cup of water to make the chia gel, set aside for at least 15 minutes.

Pre-heat oven to 180°C (350°F).

Coat baking tray with coconut oil.

Combine all ingredients together in a bowl. Mix thoroughly using your hands to roll the ingredients together.

Spread onto a baking tray and bake in the oven for 25 -30 minutes or until bread is cooked and golden brown.

While the bread is baking, prepare your chia jam.

Berry Chia Jam:

Place the berries and water in a small saucepan over medium heat and mix using a wooden spoon (using the spoon to smash the fruit as it begins to heat up and the mixture begins to boil). Continue for approximately 4 minutes.

Add the coconut nectar and chia seeds and stir through just once.

Remove the mixture from the heat, add lemon juice and cover with a cloth. Allow to sit for about 5 minutes to thicken (the chia seeds will congeal).

Once cool, transfer mixture to an airtight container and refrigerate.

Serves: 15 slices + prep: 20 min. + cook: 25-30 min.

Note

You can replace the buckwheat flour with almond flour for a Paleo-friendly version.

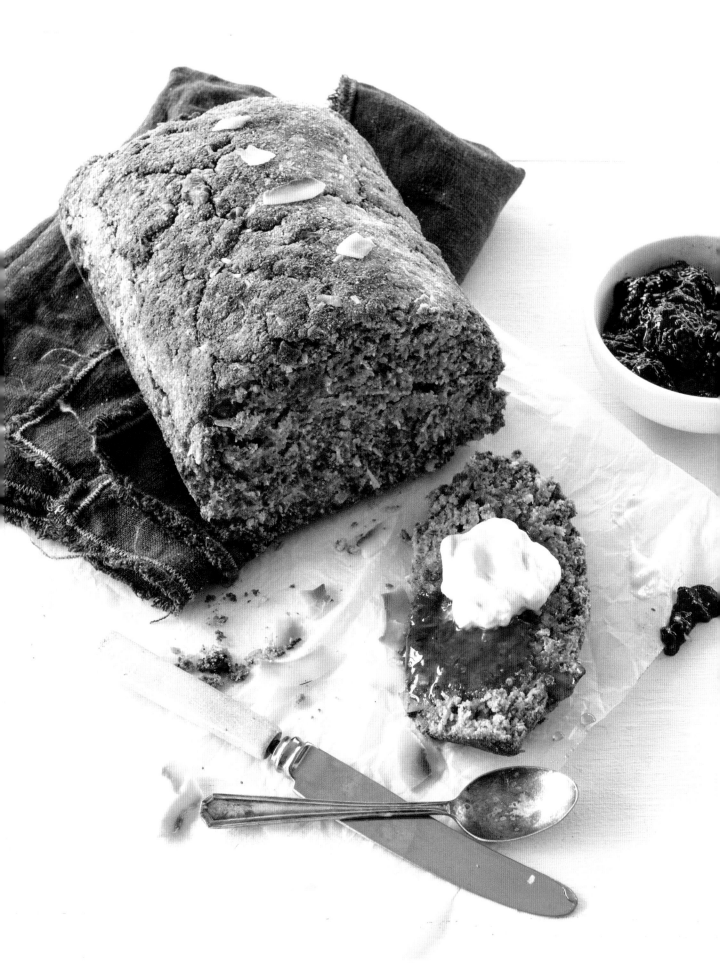

plant-based milk, cheese, butter, cream & yoghurt

plant based milks

HEMPSEED MILK

1 cup organic shelled hempseeds
(no soaking required)

3½ cups filtered or spring water

2 tbs Coconut Magic coconut oil

1 tbs Coconut Magic coconut nectar (optional)

Pinch of pink salt

Pinch of vanilla essence

Blend the hempseeds in a high-speed blender with one cup of water for 60-90 seconds, or until the hempseeds are crushed and the liquid is ultra smooth.

Strain the blended mix through a nutbag, squeezing the bag so that all of the liquid is released. If you don't have a nutbag, use a cheesecloth and a strainer. The fibre, or pulp, will remain in the nutbag – set this aside.

Pour the liquid in the bowl back into the blender and add all remaining ingredients.

Blend for just 30 seconds on low speed. We just want to mix everything together now.

Pour the fresh hempseed milk into a glass bottle and store in the fridge. Keeps refrigerated for 2-3 days.

Freeze the pulp, use it later in crackers or biscuits.

Makes 750 ml + prep: 20 min.

ALMOND MILK

1 cup organic almonds, soaked overnight

3½ cups clean water, preferably chilled

2 tbs Coconut Magic coconut oil

1 tbs Coconut Magic coconut nectar (optional)

Pinch of pink salt

Pinch of vanilla essence

Wash and rinse the soaked almonds well. Blend the almonds in a high-speed blender with one cup of water for 60-90 seconds, or until almonds are crushed and the liquid is ultra smooth.

Strain the blended mix through a nutbag, squeezing the bag so that all of the liquid is released. The fibre, or pulp, will remain in the nutbag – set this aside.

Pour the liquid in the bowl back into the blender and add all remaining ingredients.

Blend for just 30 seconds on low speed. We just want to mix everything together now.

Pour the fresh almond milk into a glass bottle and store in the fridge.

Keeps refrigerated for 2-3 days.

Makes 750 ml + prep: 20 min. + soaking: 24 hr.

Take note

Almond pulp can be used to make Bliss Balls (see page 216).

Or it can be frozen until needed.

COCONUT MILK

4 cups Coconut Magic desiccated coconut
or coconut flakes

4 cups clean water, boiled

1 pinch pink salt

Put the coconut and the water in the blender and blend until
a smooth creamy liquid forms. Add more water if required for
desired consistency.

Strain the blended mix through a nutbag, squeezing the bag
so that all of the liquid is released. If you don't have a nutbag,
use a cheesecloth and a strainer. Watch your hands as the
liquid is hot! The fibre, or pulp, will remain in the nutbag — set
this aside.

Pour the fresh coconut milk into a glass bottle, add the pinch
of salt and store in the fridge.

Freeze the pulp, use it later in crackers or biscuits.

NB: For a thinner milk consistency use an additional 1-2 cups
of clean water.

Makes approx. 1 litre + prep: 20 min.

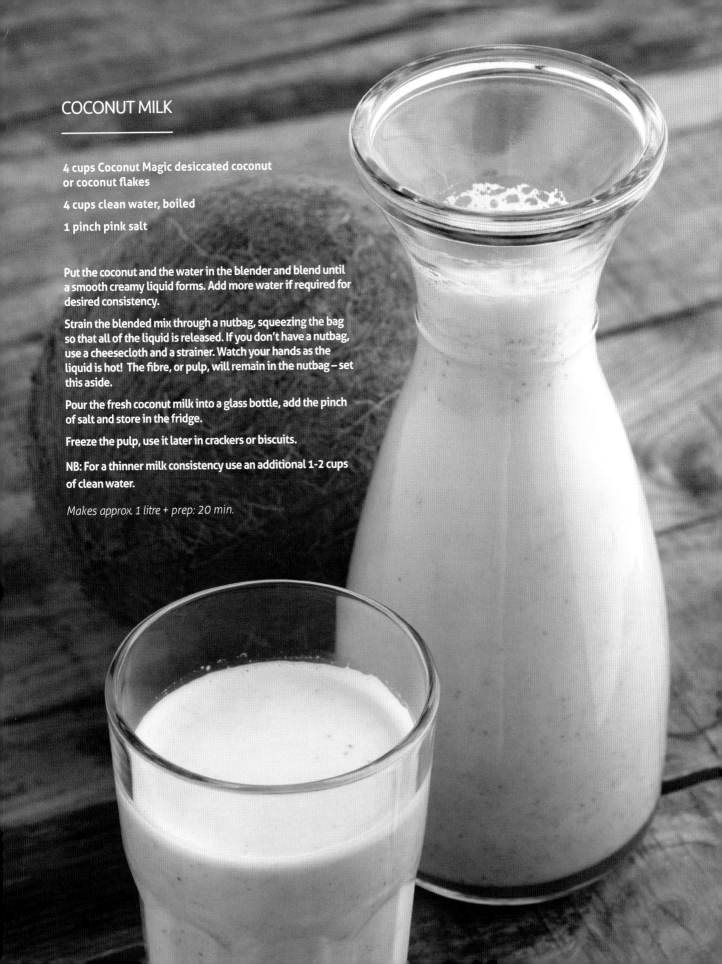

butters

CHOCOLATE BUTTER

½ cup coconut butter, melted

1 cup cashews (soaked for 2 hours)

1 tbs Coconut Magic coconut nectar

2 tbs Coconut Magic coconut oil

2 tbs cacao powder

1 tsp vanilla essence

Pinch of pink salt

In a saucepan over a low heat, slowly melt the coconut oil and coconut butter.

Transfer to a bowl and add all other ingredients and whisk until smooth.

Pour into a sealed jar and place into the fridge. The spread will solidify and the oils may separate.

May be stored at room temperature up to 3 weeks, or up to a couple of months in the refrigerator.

Makes 10-15 small serves or about 120 ml + prep: 15 min. + soaking: 2 hr.

ALMOND BUTTER

3 cups almonds (soaked overnight)

Rinse and drain the almonds in clean water. Blend almonds in a food processor, making sure the lid is tightly secured. Process for 20-30 minutes. Stop and scrape down the sides as needed.

Once the oils have released the butter becomes very smooth and creamy. This requires a little patience as it does take some time.

Transfer into a sealed glass jar and store in the fridge.

Almond butter will keep for up to two months in the fridge.

Makes 10-15 small serves + prep: 35 min. + soaking: overnight

COCONUT BUTTER

3 cups Coconut Magic desiccated coconut or coconut flakes

Blend coconut in a food processor, making sure the lid is tightly secured. Process for 10 minutes. Stop and scrape down the sides as needed.

Once the oils have released the butter becomes very smooth and creamy.

Transfer into a sealed glass jar and store at room temperature or in the fridge.

Coconut butter will keep for up to two months.

Makes 10-15 small serves + prep: 35 min. + soaking: overnight

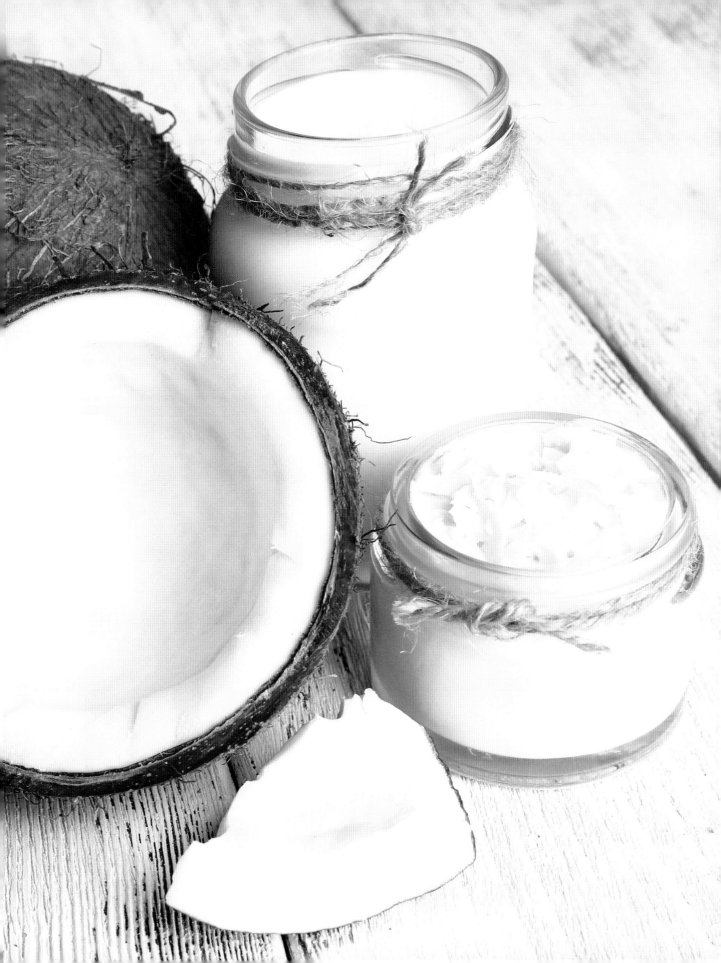

yoghurt & cream

COCONUT MILK YOGHURT

2 cups coconut milk

2 capsules probiotic powder

1 tbs Coconut Magic coconut sugar (optional)

1 tsp arrowroot powder (optional)

Warm the coconut milk in a saucepan over a low heat, until warm to touch.

Carefully pour the warm coconut milk into a sterilised jar.

Add the probiotic powder and the sweetener (if using).

Place the jar in a sunny place for 24 hours – a bench beneath a window, or on a window ledge works well. You could also place the jar in the oven with the light on.

Place the yoghurt in the fridge and then chill for a few hours.

Once stored in the fridge the yoghurt will become thicker and more tart with each passing day.

Will keep up to one week stored in the refrigerator.

Serves 6-8 + prep: 25 min. Fermentation: 24 hr.

CASHEW YOGHURT

2 cups raw cashews, soaked overnight

2 cups clean water

2 tbs Coconut Magic coconut nectar

2 capsules probiotic powder

Pinch of pink salt

1 tsp vanilla essence

Drain and rinse the soaked cashews.

Add all ingredients to a high-speed blender and blend until the mixture is completely smooth and there are no lumps remaining.

Transfer the mixture into a bowl and cover with a cheesecloth or a tea towel.

Leave the bowl and mixture in a warm place for 24-36 hours. It will start to become tangy and develop a strong but pleasant smell. The longer you leave it, the tangier it becomes.

When the yoghurt has fermented, give it a good stir. Transfer into a well-sealed jar or a container.

Will keep up to one week in your fridge.

Serves 6-8 + prep: 25 min. Fermentation: 24 hr.

Take note

For best results your probiotic powder must contain one of these strains – Lactobacillus bulgaricus, Streptococcus thermophilus, Bifidobacterium lactis or Lactobacillus acidophilus.

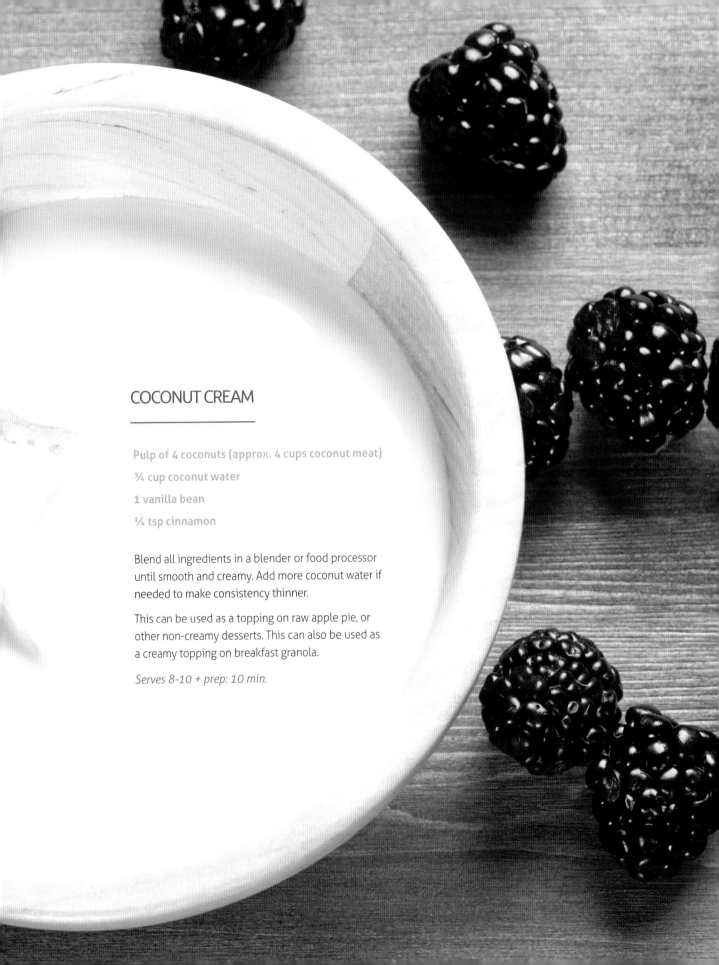

COCONUT CREAM

Pulp of 4 coconuts (approx. 4 cups coconut meat)

¾ cup coconut water

1 vanilla bean

¼ tsp cinnamon

Blend all ingredients in a blender or food processor until smooth and creamy. Add more coconut water if needed to make consistency thinner.

This can be used as a topping on raw apple pie, or other non-creamy desserts. This can also be used as a creamy topping on breakfast granola.

Serves 8-10 + prep: 10 min.

nut cheeses

These are healthy alternatives to dairy-based cheeses, and are simple to make!

EASY CASHEW CHEESE

2 cups cashews, soaked for 2 hours

2 tbs olive oil

2-3 tbs lemon juice

1 tsp pink salt

1 tsp granulated garlic

1 tbs Coconut Magic coconut nectar

½ cup fresh basil leaves (optional)

Fresh cracked black pepper, to taste

Blend all ingredients in a high-speed blender using a tamper to assist. Start at a slow speed and slowly build up until the ingredients become creamy. You might need to stop along the way to scrape down the sides.

Add more olive oil and lemon juice if required to achieve the desired consistency.

Transfer the cheese into a glass jar or container and seal.

Serves 12+ prep: 15 min. soaking: 2 hr.

MACADAMIA CREAM CHEESE

1 cup macadamias

½ cup cashew nuts (soaked for 2 hours)

2 tbs lime juice

1 tbs red onion, chopped

1 tsp cumin powder

1 tsp pink salt

½ cup clean water

Pinch cayenne pepper

2 tbs olive oil

Blend all together until creamy. Store in the fridge.

Serves 12+ prep: 25 min. soaking: 2 hr.

Take note

You can use basil, dill or parsley for a variety of herb flavours.

Toss with zucchini noodles, spread on crackers, eat as a dip with carrots and celery, or use as a topping with your favourite raw or grain-free pizza recipe on page 140.

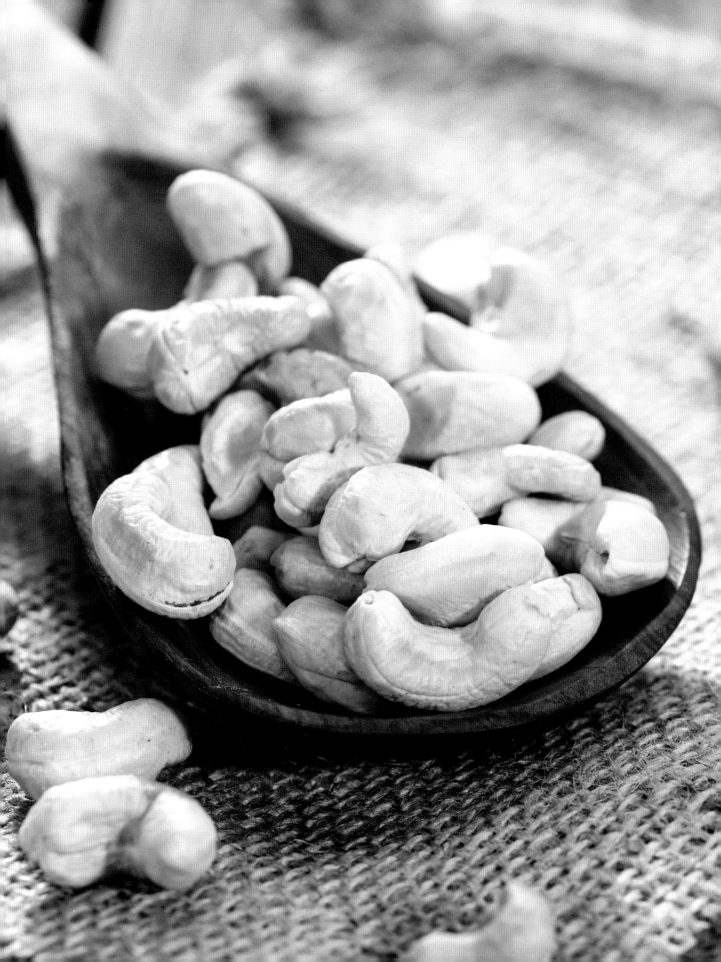

soups

CARROT, GINGER AND SWEET POTATO SOUP

8 carrots

3 tbs Coconut Magic coconut oil

2 tbs Coconut Magic coconut nectar

1 large sweet potato, peeled
and chopped

1 tsp sweet paprika

Pinch cayenne pepper (optional)

1 onion, diced

3 tbs ginger, grated

2 cloves garlic, minced

1 tsp curry powder

1 tsp cumin

6 cups clean water

1½ tbs miso paste

Preheat oven to 180°C (350°F).

Coat carrots in coconut oil and coconut nectar and roast in
the oven for 40 minutes.

Coat sweet potato in paprika, cayenne pepper and coconut
oil, roast in the oven for 30 minutes.

Fry onion, garlic and ginger together in a large saucepan for
5 minutes, or until the onion becomes translucent.

Add curry powder and cumin to onions and mix together for
one minute.

Add water, vegetables and miso paste and simmer for 10
minutes.

Allow the stock to cool a little and then blend in a blender
until smooth and creamy.

Garnish with chili flakes and green onion.

Serves 4 + prep: 60 min.

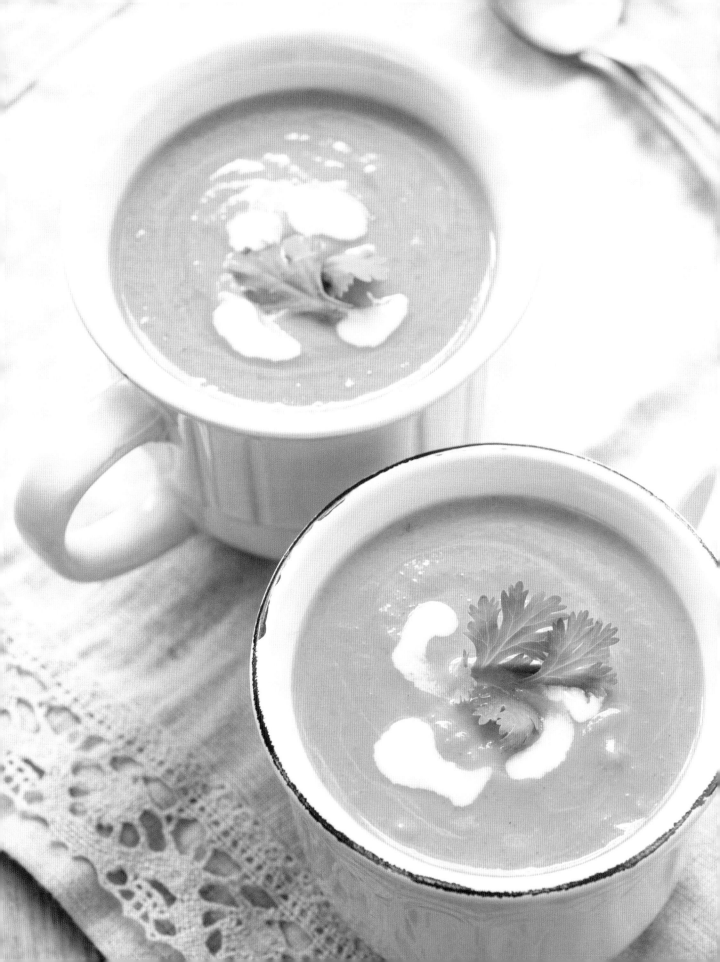

PUMPKIN SOUP

1 large butternut pumpkin peeled and chopped into small pieces

1 large onion, diced

3 tbs Coconut Magic coconut oil

1 tbs fresh ginger, chopped

1 tsp cumin

1 tsp turmeric

1 tsp curry powder, to taste

2 tsp pink salt

4-6 cups of clean water

Coconut cream to garnish

⅓ toasted Coconut Magic coconut flakes to garnish

In a large pot, fry the onion in the coconut oil for a minute.

Add all of the spices and stir for one minute.

Add water and pumpkin.

Allow the water to come to a boil, then reduce heat and simmer for 20 minutes, or until pumpkin is soft.

Using a stick blender, or transfer into food processor (you may need to do this in batches), blend until creamy and smooth.

Serve into soup bowls and add a dollop of coconut yoghurt and parsley to garnish.

Serves 4-6 + prep: 25 min.

LEMON LENTIL SOUP

3 tbs Coconut Magic coconut oil

1 large onion

3 cloves garlic

1 tsp cumin powder

1½ cups red lentils , washed

4 - 6 cups clean water

1½ tbs miso paste

1 tsp pink salt

1 cup cabbage, chopped

1 small bunch of kale, stems removed and washed

1 large lemon juiced

Coriander to garnish, chopped finely

Dulse flakes for garnish

Heat coconut oil in a large pan over low-to-medium heat. Add onion, garlic and cumin powder and cook for 2-3 minutes as the onion browns. Add water and miso paste, then the lentils.

Allow the water to come to the boil, then cover and simmer for 15-20 minutes. The lentils will start to become tender and thicken the soup.

Keep adding water – the lentils will continue to absorb the liquid.

Add salt and cabbage and cook for another 5-10 minutes. Stir in kale and lemon juice.

Serve in large soup bowls with a sprinkle of coriander and dulse flakes.

Add lemon juice and dulse flakes to taste.

Serves 4-6+ prep: 30 min.

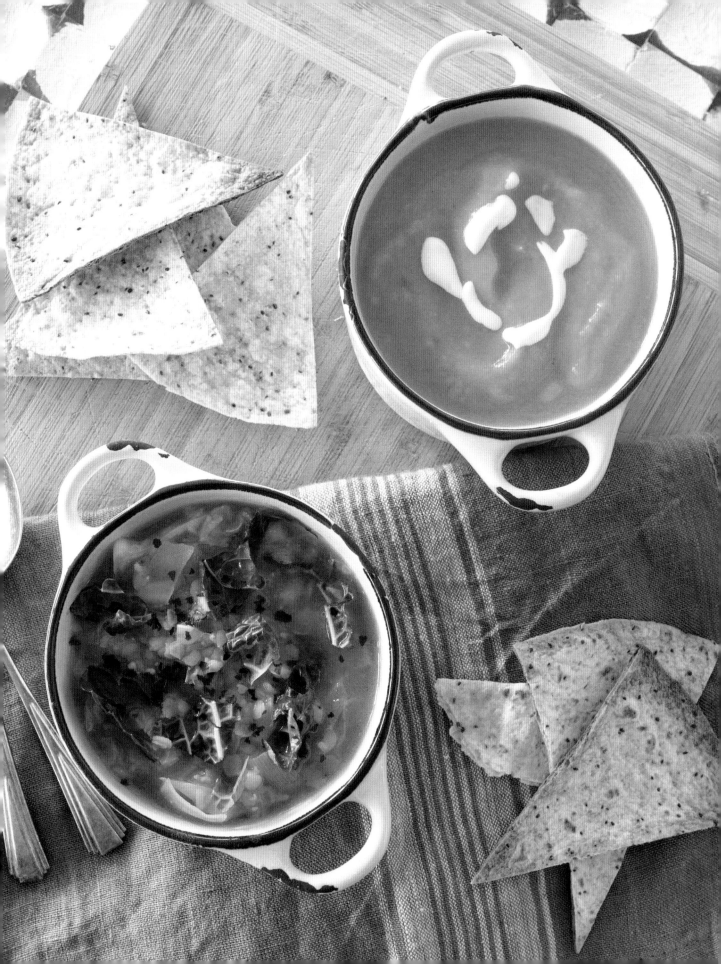

THAI STYLE COCONUT & VEGETABLE SOUP

1 brown onion, finely sliced

2 tbs Coconut Magic coconut oil

3 kaffir lime leaves, sliced

1 stalk lemongrass, sliced

1 small piece of fresh ginger, grated

½ inch piece turmeric, grated
– or ½ teaspoon turmeric powder

½ red chili – or as hot as you like it

¼ cup basil leaves

1 lime zest and juice

1½ cups coconut milk

2 tbs coconut amino or tamari sauce

2 cups of clean water

VEGETABLES

200g snow peas, julienned
(sliced very fine)

1 cup sweet potato, sliced into small
thin slices

1 bunch of bok choy, chopped finely

½ bunch of coriander

Saute the onions in the coconut oil until soft.

Add the kaffir lime leaves, lemongrass, ginger, chili, turmeric, lime zest. Cook for a further 5 minutes stirring regularly.

Add coconut milk, sweet potato and water. Simmer gently with the lid on for 15 minutes allowing the flavours to blend into the soup.

Add the tamari sauce, snow peas, bok choy, basil leaves and lime juice and stir.

Simmer for a further 5 minutes, add half the coriander, and then remove from heat.

Garnish with the remaining coriander and serve.

Serves 4 + prep: 30 min.

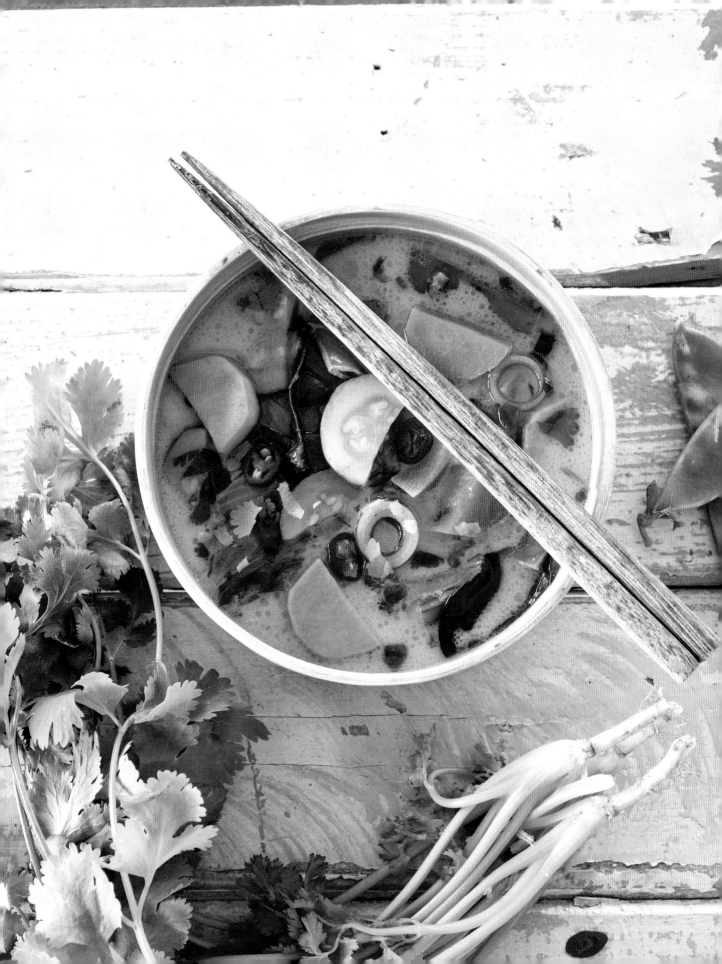

ROASTED EGGPLANT SOUP

1 large eggplant

4 large tomatoes

3 cloves garlic

1 brown onion, chopped

3 tbs Coconut Magic coconut oil (melted)

2 celery stalks, chopped

1 litre water

2 tbs miso paste

2 tsp thyme

Preheat the oven to 200°C (400°F).

Slice the eggplant in half, leaving the skin on.

Wash the tomatoes and remove the green stems from the tops. Peel the garlic.

Coat a medium-sized baking dish with coconut oil. Add the eggplant, garlic and tomatoes to the dish. Cover the top of the vegetables with more of the coconut oil, and roast for approximately 40 minutes.

While the vegetables are roasting, put the water and the rest of the ingredients into a large pot. Bring to the boil and then simmer for about 25 minutes, or until the roasted vegetables are ready.

Remove the vegetables from the oven and, taking care not to burn your hands, chop the eggplant and tomato into medium-sized chunks.

Add the roasted vegetables, eggplant, tomato, onion and garlic to the pot. Leave on a low flame for 5-10 minutes allowing the flavours to integrate. Allow to cool slightly.

Using a stick blender or food processor, blend until smooth.

Serves 4 - 6 + prep: 15 min.

GREEN DETOX SOUP

1 large onion, chopped

1 large broccoli, broken into florets

1 small sweet potato, peeled and chopped

2 zucchini, chopped

½ cauliflower, diced

2 stalks of celery, chopped into small pieces

1 cup fresh parsley, chopped

¼ cup of sweet basil

2 cloves garlic

6-8 cups of clean water

Pink salt and nutritional yeast to taste

Olive oil and parsley to garnish

Place onion, sweet potato, and water in a large pot of water and bring to the boil. Add broccoli, cauliflower, zucchini and celery. Leave over medium heat for 10 minutes then allow to cool.

Place the garlic and parsley inside the blender. Add the vegetables and the broth to the blender and blend all together until smooth. You may need to do this in batches, depending on volume.

Add pink salt to taste.

Serve into soup bowls and top with a little olive oil and nutritional yeast for added flavor.

Serves 4 + prep: 20 min.

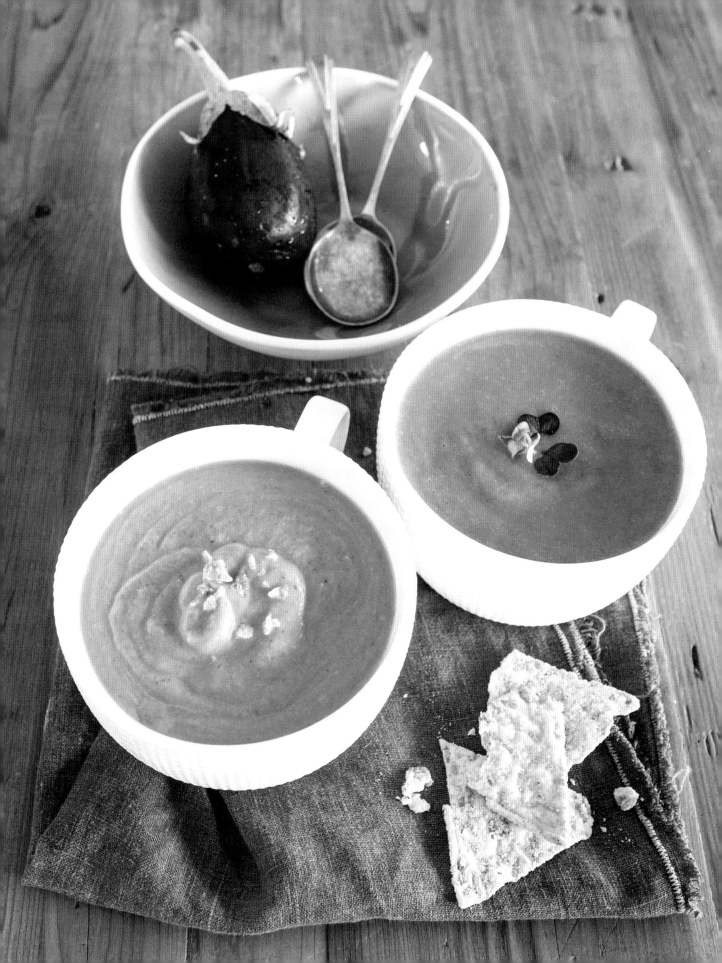

RAW TOM YUM SOUP

1 cup coconut meat
(from a young Thai coconut)

2 cups coconut water

1 whole lemongrass stalk

1 small piece of ginger

1 small clove garlic

3 tbs sweet basil

3 tbs parsley

1 bunch coriander

2 tbs lime juice

1 tsp Italian seasoning

1 tbs olive oil

1 tbs Coconut Magic coconut oil

½ tsp pink salt

1 tbs coconut aminos or tamari sauce

Blend all ingredients in a high-speed blender until smooth.

This is a very full-flavoured dish!

Serves 4 small or 2 large bowls + prep: 20 min.

RAW COCONUT SOUP

BROTH

2 cups coconut meat

1½ cups coconut water

1 small clove garlic (optional)

1 tbs fresh minced ginger

3 tbs lime juice

2 tbs Coconut Magic coconut oil

2 tbs fresh coriander, chopped

¼ tsp pink salt

Pinch cayenne pepper (optional)

GARNISH

1 tomato

½ red capsicum, sliced

4-5 button mushrooms to garnish

Open the coconut and drain the coconut water into a blender.

Scrape out the flesh and add to blender.

Add remaining broth ingredients and blend into liquid consistency.

Divide evenly into two serving bowls.

Add any chopped veggies that you like to the bowls: bell pepper, tomatoes and thinly sliced mushrooms work well.

Serves 2 large bowls + prep: 20 min.

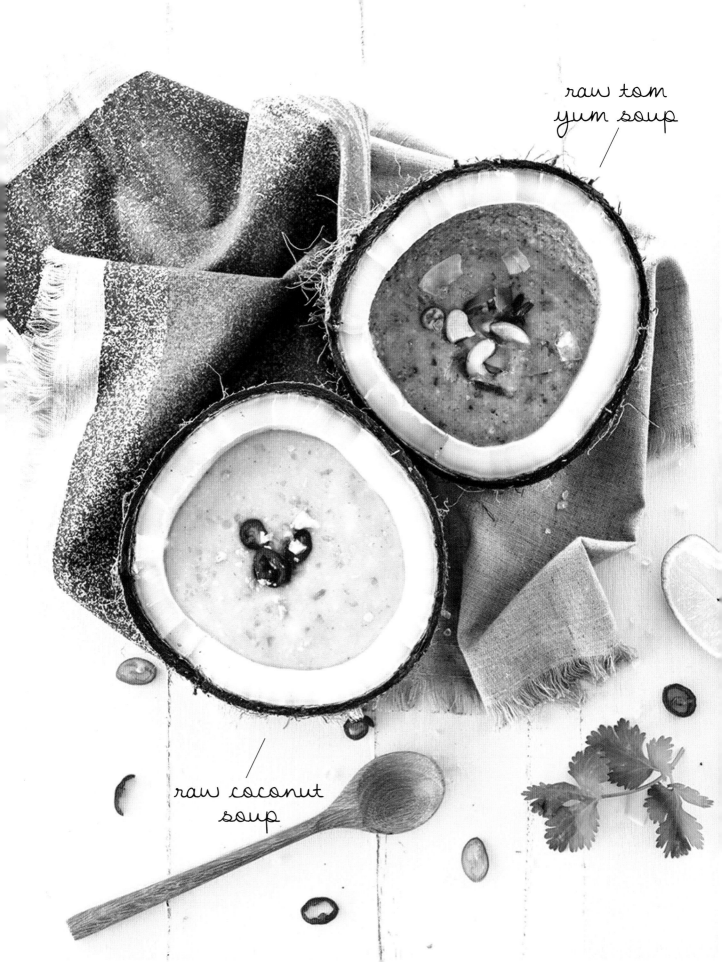

raw tom yum soup

raw coconut soup

CREAMY TOMATO BASIL SOUP

1 organic red pepper, cored, deseeded and chopped

3 medium-sized, organic vine-ripened tomatoes

1 organic celery stalk chopped fine

½ cup coconut flesh (or coconut milk)

¼ cup chopped white onion

1 tbs nutritional yeast

¾ tsp pink salt

1 very small garlic clove (optional)

1 tbs fresh lemon juice

2 tbs Coconut Magic coconut oil

¼ cup fresh basil leaves

Blend everything until smooth and serve.

If you'd like to warm it gently, blend for longer, or warm it over the stove on the lowest temperature, but don't bring to a boil or overheat.

Serves 4 + prep: 10 min.

RAW AVOCADO & CUCUMBER SOUP

2 whole cucumbers

2 whole large avocados

2 cups coconut water

2 tbs lime juice

1 tbs dill

1 tbs olive oil

1 small tomato, chopped finely

Pinch of pink salt

Pinch of pepper

1 tsp desiccated coconut, unsweetened

Blend in a high-speed blender until smooth. Add more lemon or lime juice to suit your taste.

Garnish with some fresh unsweetened desiccated coconut.

Serves 4 + prep: 10 min.

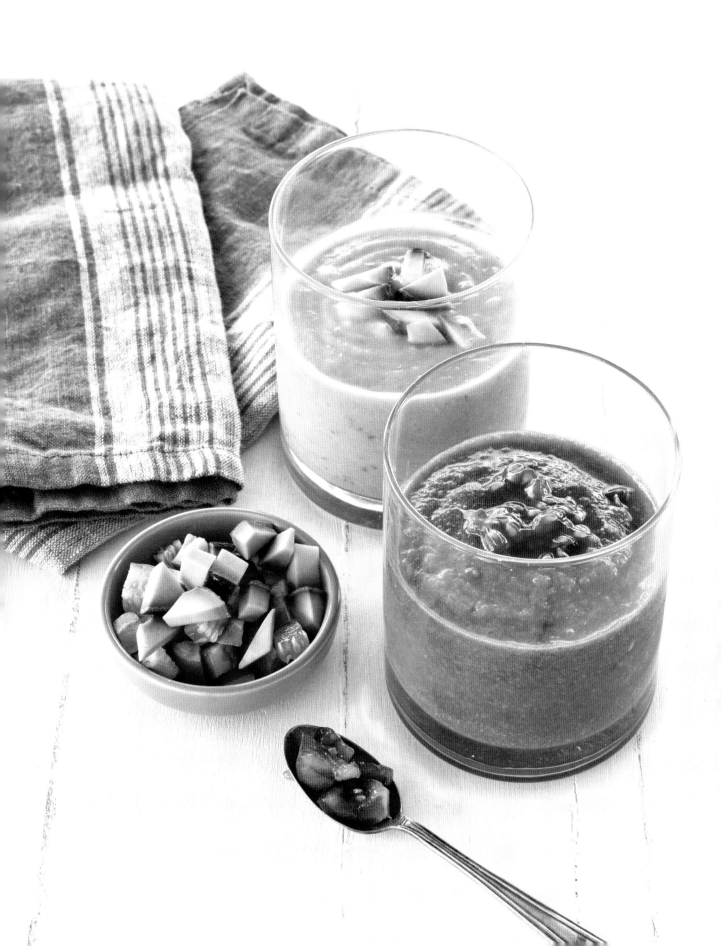

main meals

VEGAN MOUSSAKA

VEGGIES

1 large eggplant, sliced lengthways into ¼ thick inch slices, covered with salt and set aside

2 large zucchini

2 medium sweet potatoes

¼ cup Coconut Magic coconut oil (melted)

1 cup rice-crumbs

TOMATO SAUCE

2 tbs Coconut Magic coconut oil

1 white onion, chopped finely

3 cloves garlic, minced

⅓ cup vegetable broth

6 large soft tomatoes, crushed

2 tsp dried oregano

¼ tsp cinnamon

1 tsp tomato paste

1 bay leaf

½ tsp Coconut Magic coconut sugar

Pinch of pink salt, to taste

NUT CHEESE TOPPING

1 cup cashews, soaked

1 cup pine nuts

4 tbs lemon juice

1 tsp arrowroot powder

1 clove of garlic

½ teaspoon nutmeg

1 tsp pink salt to taste

Pepper to taste

2 tbs clean water

Vegetables: Preheat oven to 200°C (400°F). Lightly oil 3 baking sheets/dishes. Peel the potatoes and slice both zucchini and potatoes in the same way. Rinse the eggplant and pat dry. Place each of the vegetables on their own baking sheet. Sprinkle the ¼ cup of melted coconut oil over the vegetables, making sure that all the veggies are coated (use your hands to cover them well). Sprinkle the zucchini and potato with salt. Roast the vegetables, approximately 15 minutes for the eggplant and zucchini, and 20 minutes for the sweet potato.

Tomato sauce: Fry the coconut oil, garlic and onion in a pan over a medium heat for about 3 minutes, or until onions are browned and garlic is soft. Add in the crushed tomatoes, vegetable broth and tomato paste. Mix well. Add the coconut sugar, oregano, cinnamon and bay leaf. Leave covered and simmer for about 20 minutes.

Add some clean water if required, so the mixture stays moist. The sauce will thicken and reduce.

After cooking, adjust the salt to taste and remove the bay leaf.

Nut cheese: Using a food processor blend the cashew nuts and the pine nuts and lemon juice into a paste. Add the garlic, arrowroot, nutmeg, salt and pepper and blend for approximately 3 minutes, or until creamy and smooth. Add some clean water as required for a softer consistency.

Putting it all together: Lightly oil a 9 x 13 inch casserole dish. Preheat oven to 200°C. (400°F). Spread about ½ cup of the tomato sauce at the bottom of the dish, followed by a layer of eggplant, a layer of potatoes, a layer of tomato sauce and half of the rice-crumbs. Follow with another sequence of the eggplant, potato, tomato layer as above, with some more rice-crumbs. The next layer uses all the zucchini. Top with another layer of eggplant, potato and tomato and the remainder of the rice-crumbs. Spread the nut cheese on last, using a spatula to spread it out as best you can without disturbing the layers underneath.

Bake the Moussaka for 40 minutes until the top is lightly browned and a few cracks start to form in the topping. Allow to set for 10 minutes before slicing and serving.

Serves 6-8 + prep: 1 hr + cook: 40 min.

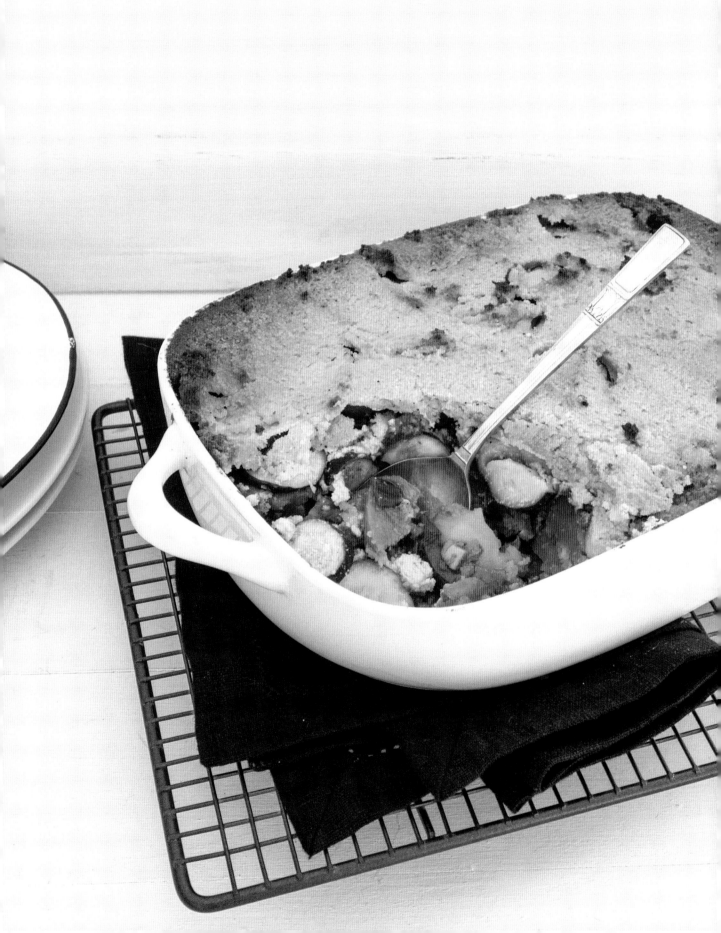

COCONUT LENTIL CURRY WITH CAULIFLOWER RICE

THE COCONUT LENTIL CURRY

¼ cup Coconut Magic coconut oil

1 white onion, chopped

4 cloves garlic, minced

5 large ripe tomatoes

2 cups clean water

1-2 tbs curry powder (depending on how spicy you like it!)

1½ cups coconut milk

1 tbs Coconut Magic coconut nectar

2 tbs ground coriander

1 tbs cinnamon powder

2 cups red lentils, washed and rinsed

1 bunch fresh parsley, washed and chopped

Pink salt and black pepper, to taste

CAULIFLOWER RICE

1 cauliflower, florets and stalk roughly chopped

2 tbs Coconut Magic coconut oil

Pink salt and black pepper, to taste

The Lentil Curry:

Melt the coconut oil in a large pan over medium heat. Sauté the onions and garlic until tender, about 5 minutes.

Add the tomatoes and cook for 5 more minutes.

Add in the water, curry powder, coconut milk, coconut nectar, ground coriander and cinnamon.

Stir in the lentils and allow them to cook for 10-15 minutes, they will become tender as they absorb the liquid. Stir frequently and enjoy the aroma as the curry becomes fragrant.

Once the lentils have become soft, stir in the pink salt, pepper and parsley.

The Cauliflower Rice:

Pulse the cauliflower in a food processor – you want it to end up looking like rice.

Fry cauliflower with some coconut oil over medium heat for approximately 5 minutes, or until softened.

Season with salt and pepper and serve. Serve with a garden or Greek salad.

Serves 4 - 6 + prep: 15 min. + cook: 25 min.

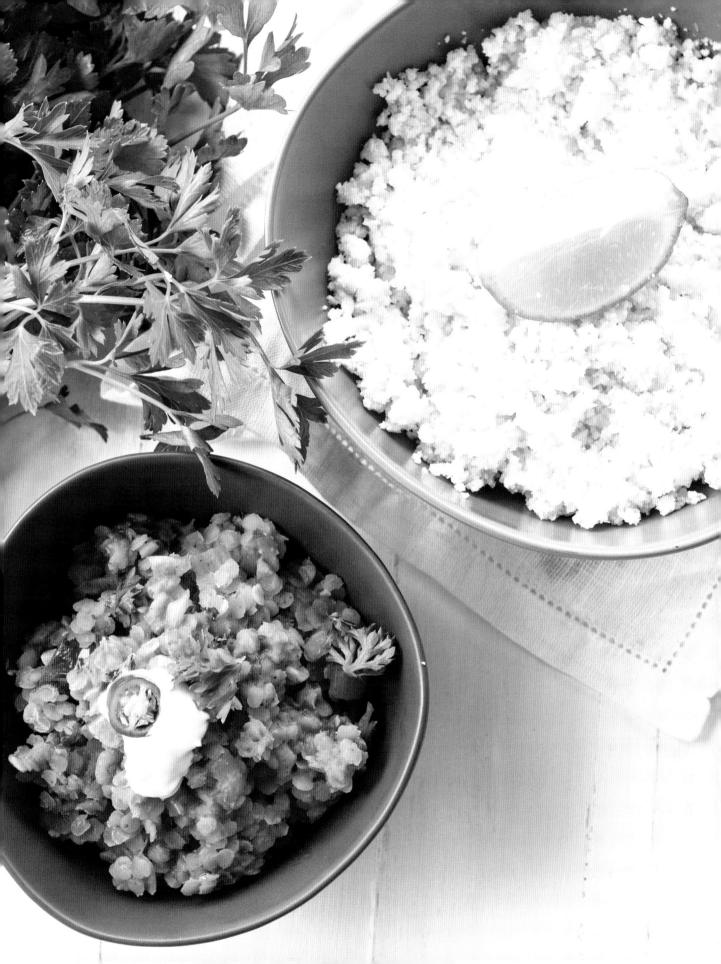

FALAFELS WITH TAHINI YOGHURT

FALAFELS

2 cups dried chickpeas, soaked overnight in a large bowl filled with clean water

1 onion, chopped

4-5 cloves of garlic, peeled and roughly chopped

1 cup fresh parsley

2 tsp pink salt

Pepper to taste

1 tbs coriander

½ tsp cayenne pepper

2 tsp cumin powder

3 tbs chickpea flour

1 tsp baking soda (aluminium free)

½ tsp baking powder

¾ cup Coconut Magic coconut oil for frying

TAHINI YOGHURT

½ cup plain coconut yogurt

¼ cup tahini

1 tbs lemon juice

1 clove garlic, minced (optional)

2 tbs coriander freshly chopped

Falafels:

Drain the chickpeas and pulse in a food processor until crumbly and no whole chickpeas are left. Transfer to a large bowl and set aside.

In the same food processor, pulse together the onion, garlic, parsley and coriander, until it almost looks like a paste.

Add parsley mixture to chickpeas, then add cumin, cayenne, salt, pepper and chickpea flour. Mix well.

Add baking powder and baking soda at the last minute before frying. Mix everything well.

Heat the coconut oil in a large fry pan until it is hot. You can test to see if the oil is hot by dropping in a small piece of batter. If it sizzles, it's ready.

Use a large tablespoon and form batter into balls. Scoop about 2 tablespoons' worth and form a ball between your hands. The falafel balls might seem soft but they will harden once they are in the oil.

Carefully place the falafel in the hot oil. You can fit 4-5 in at once.

Brown one side, for about 3-4 minutes, then flip over and fry the other side. The falafel should be crisp on the outside and soft on the inside.

Tahini Yoghurt:

Blend all ingredients in a small mixer or blender until smooth.

Serve with hempseed tabouli salad, page 180.

Serves 6-8 + prep: 1 hr. + cook: 40 min.

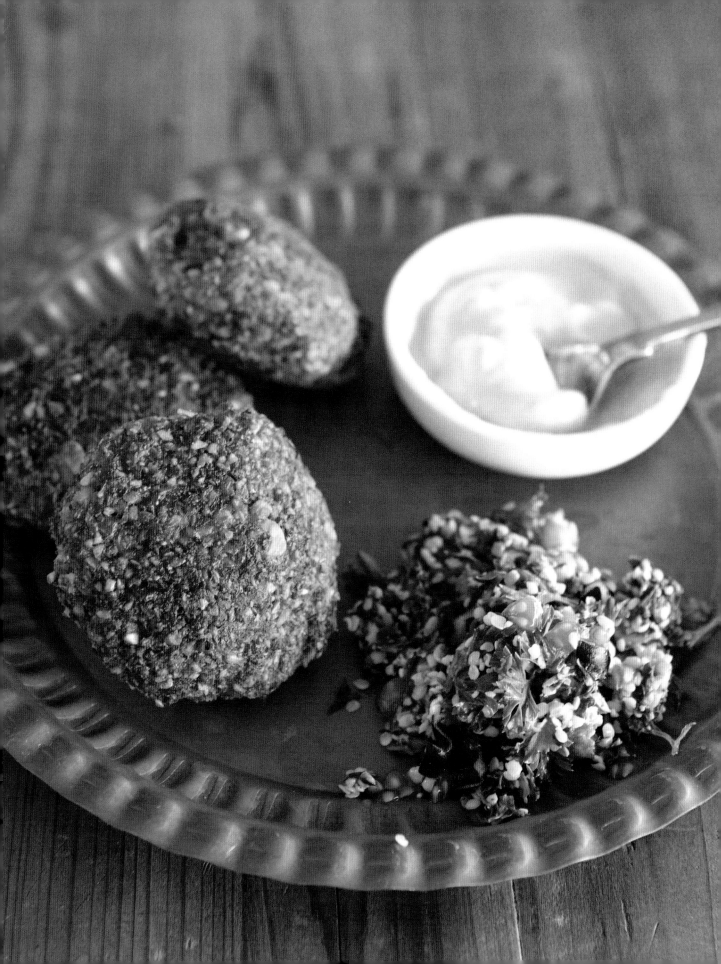

COCONUT QUINOA WITH KALE & PESTO

COCONUT QUINOA

1 cup coconut milk (to make your own, see recipe on page 109)

1 cup clean water

1 cup quinoa, rinsed well

1 small bunch of kale, stems removed and leaves chopped (for a total of about 4 cups chopped kale)

½ small-to-medium red onion, chopped

2 cups Coconut Magic coconut flakes

BASIL PESTO

2 cups fresh basil leaves, packed

½ cup cashews

2-3 cloves garlic

½ cup olive oil

Pink salt and black pepper, to taste

½ lime, juiced (or more, to taste)

Pinch red pepper flakes, optional

The Quinoa:

In a medium saucepan, combine 1 cup coconut milk and 1 cup clean water, and bring to the boil.

Add the quinoa, cover and simmer for 15 to 17 minutes, until the filtered water is absorbed.

Remove from heat, fluff with a fork, cover and set aside.

The Pesto:

Combine the fresh basil, cashews and garlic in a food processor.

Start processing the mixture, and slowly drizzle in the olive oil.

Season with salt, pepper, lime juice and red pepper flakes, all to taste, and blend well.

In a medium serving bowl, combine the warm coconut quinoa, chopped kale, red onion and pesto.

Mix well with a big spoon and season to taste with salt and pepper, if necessary.

Serves 4-6 + prep: 30 min. + cook: 25 - 30 min.

Optional

In a skillet over medium heat, toast the coconut flakes for a few minutes until golden and fragrant, stirring often.

Sprinkle on top of the salad and serve warm.

You can also replace the basil with coriander for a beautiful coriander pesto option.

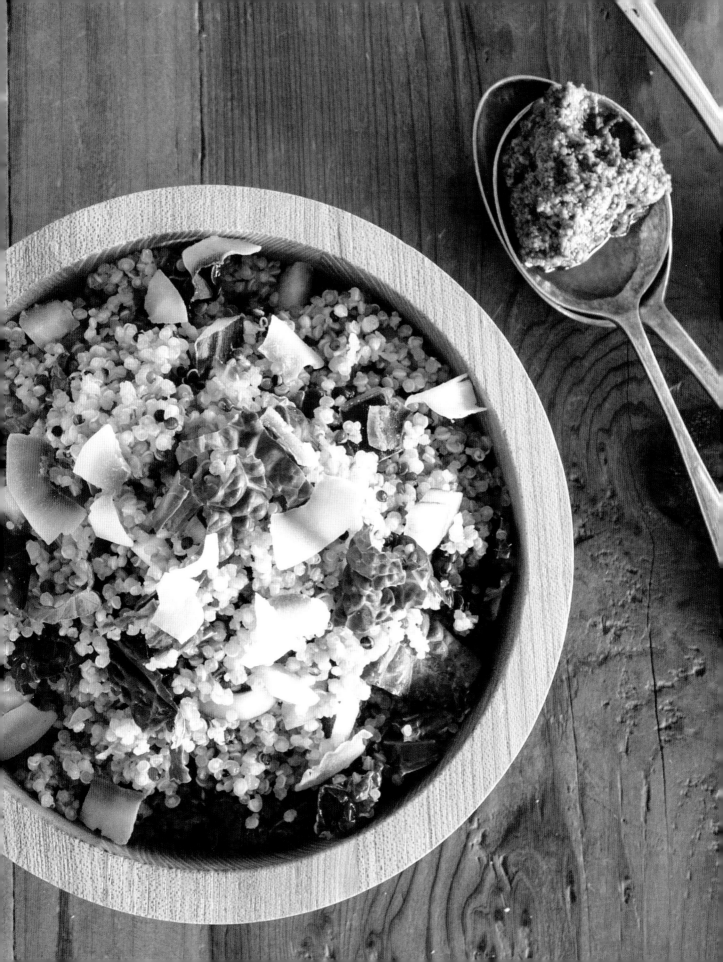

GRAIN-FREE VEGETABLE PIZZA

PIZZA BASE

½ cup ground flax seed

1 cup of clean water

3 cups cauliflower florets

1½ cups almond meal

½ tsp garlic powder

½ tsp dried oregano

2 tbs Coconut Magic coconut oil

CASHEW PARMESAN

½ cup cashews

¼ cup clean water

1 tsp nutritional yeast

Pink salt and pepper, to taste

TOPPING OPTIONS

Sundried tomatoes, diced

Spinach leaves

Kalamata olives, diced

Red onion, sliced

Mushrooms, sliced

Capsicum, sliced

Tomato, sliced

Rocket leaves

Pizza Base:

Preheat the oven to 200°C (400°F).

Line a baking tray with baking paper.

Place the flax seeds in a bowl with one cup of filtered water to make 'flax eggs' and set aside for 15 minutes.

Add cauliflower to food processor and pulse until a rice-like texture is formed.

Place the riced cauliflower in a bowl and add all other ingredients, including the flax eggs.

Scoop this mix onto the lined baking tray, to the desired thickness.

Bake in the oven for 25-30 minutes.

Prepare your topping ingredients and add to the pizza.

Cashew Parmesan:

In a small food processor, combine all of the ingredients and process until a crumbly, uniform texture is created. Feel free to adjust the flavor to your taste.

Pour over the pizza toppings.

Return to the oven for another 10 minutes, or until the 'cheese' turns slightly brown.

Slice and serve.

Makes 6 large slices + prep: 40 min. + cook: 30 min.

> ## Note
>
> For more cheese topping recipe options see page 114.

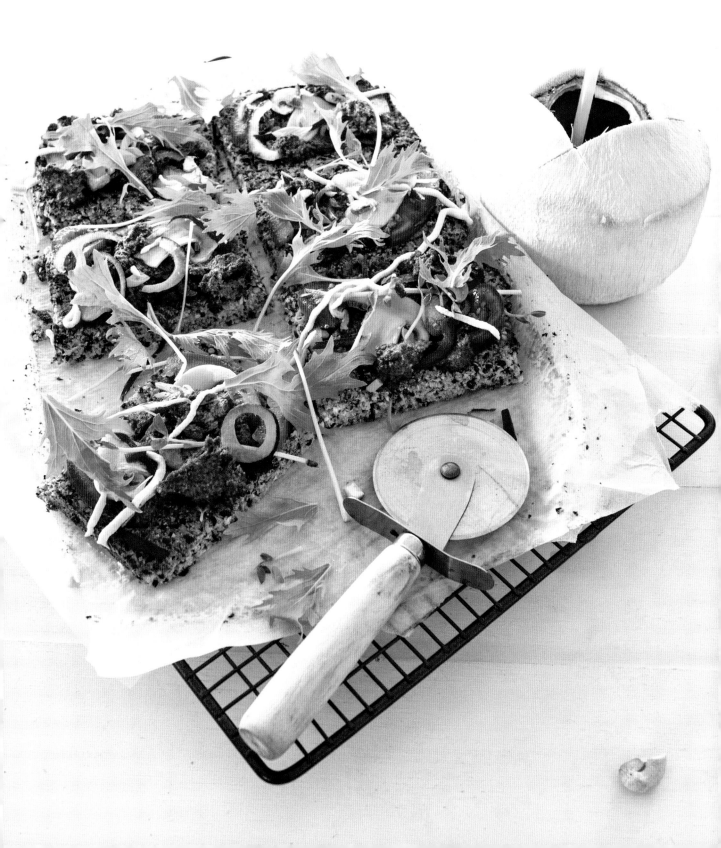

ROASTED VEGETABLES IN COCONUT MAGIC COCONUT OIL

1 bunch baby carrots, whole

3 small sweet potatoes cut into large pieces

4 small white potatoes cut into large pieces

2 onions, whole or cut into half

2 beetroots, whole

6-8 small parsnips, whole

½ cup Coconut Magic coconut oil, melted

2 tsp Italian herbs or rosemary

Pink salt, to taste

2 tsp Coconut Magic coconut nectar

Preheat oven to 200°C (400°F).

Coat the bottom of a large baking pan with coconut oil.

Place all of vegetables in the pan and drizzle coconut oil over the top making sure that all veggies are covered.

Drizzle the coconut nectar over the carrots.

Sprinkle the herbs and salt over the top.

Bake in the oven for about 40 minutes. At the halfway point, gently move the vegetables with a wooden spatula, to ensure they are moist and covered in coconut oil.

Once the potatoes are starting to brown, remove from the oven and serve.

Serves 4-6 + prep: 15 min. + cook: 40 min.

Optional

You can use a variety of vegetables for the dish. Pumpkin, sweed and zucchini all work really well too. Make your own roast vegetable combo!

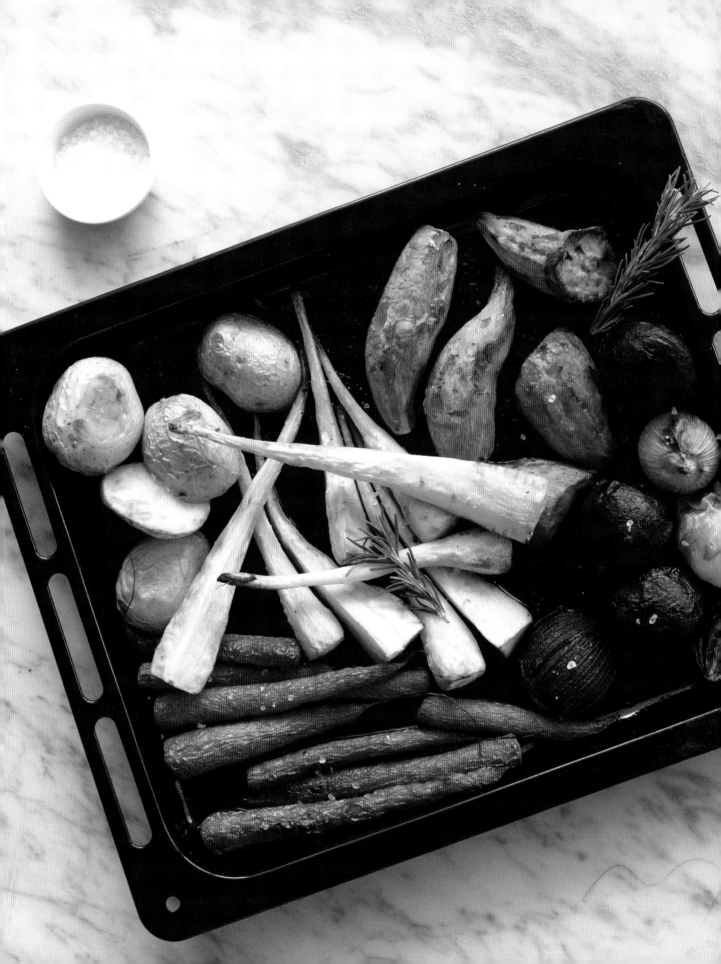

RAW ZUCCHINI PASTA WITH BASIL SAUCE

PASTA

3 zucchini, ends trimmed

1 cup spinach leaves

12 Kalamata olives, pitted

12 cherry tomatoes, halved

½ cup hemp seeds

Pink salt to taste

1 sliced green spring onion to serve

Lemon wedges to serve

BASIL SAUCE

½ cup basil leaves

½ cup olive oil

½ cup raw cashews

1 small piece of garlic

2 tbs lemon juice

2 tbs Coconut Magic coconut vinegar

1 tsp Coconut Magic coconut nectar

Pink salt, to taste

Pasta:

Using a spiraliser slice the zucchini into noodles. (You can use a vegetable peeler if you don't have a spiraliser.)

In a bowl, add the noodles to the spinach leaves, olives and tomatoes. Set aside.

Basil Sauce:

Place all ingredients into a small mixer or blender and blend until a smooth consistency is achieved.

Pour the dressing over the zucchini noodles using just enough to cover all of the vegetables.

Sprinkle the hemp seeds over the top of the noodles and stir the hemp seeds and the dressing through the salad.

Garnish with spring onion and lemon wedges.

Serves 4 + prep: 20 min.

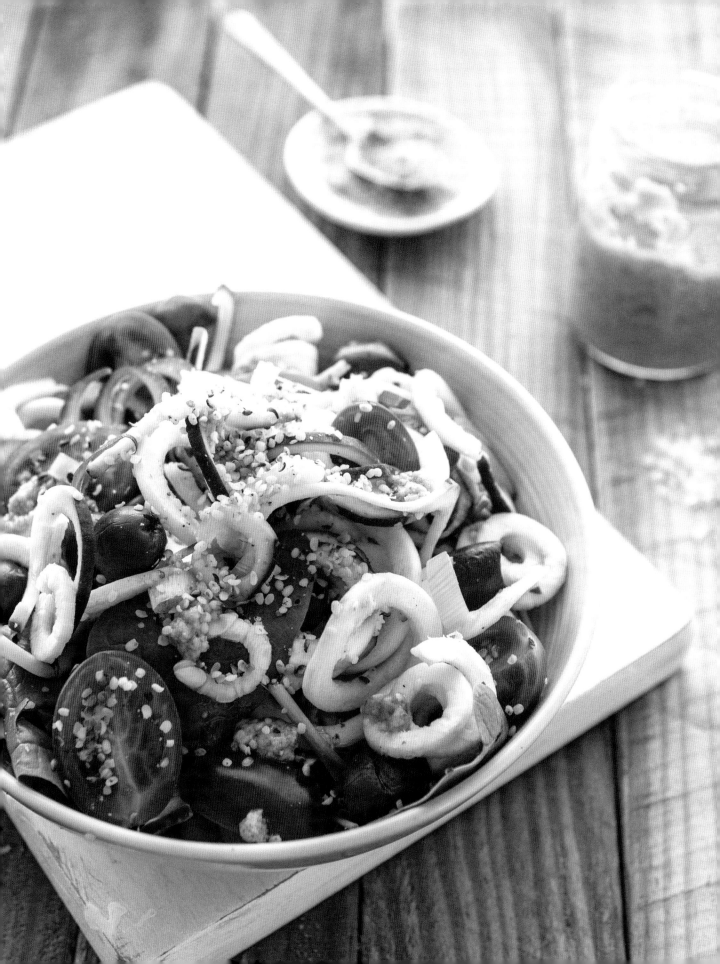

RAW SOFT TACOS WITH WALNUT MEAT

WALNUT MEAT

3 cups walnuts, ground

1 tsp cumin powder

1 tsp coriander seed powder

⅓ cup namu shoyu or tamari sauce

TOMATO SALSA

1 cup of tomatoes, chopped

1 red onion, chopped

2 tbs lemon juice

1 small red bell pepper, chopped

1 cup coriander, stems removed and chopped finely

¼ cup olive oil

½ tsp garlic, minced (optional)

Pinch cayenne pepper, to taste (optional)

Pinch of pink salt

1 tsp cumin powder

MACADAMIA CREAM CHEESE

(see page 114)

TACO SHELL

Collard green leaves

TOPPING

1 avocado, cubed

Black sesame seeds to garnish

Walnut Meat:

To make the filling, combine all Walnut Meat ingredients in a bowl and mix well.

Tomato Salsa:

In another bowl, combine the Salsa ingredients and mix well.

To Assemble:

Lay the green leaves flat. Spread the taco filling lengthwise. Top with tomato salsa and cubed avocado.

Drizzle the macadamia cream cheese over the top of the tacos.

Garnish with black sesame seeds and lemon wedges.

Serves 4-6 + prep: 25 min.

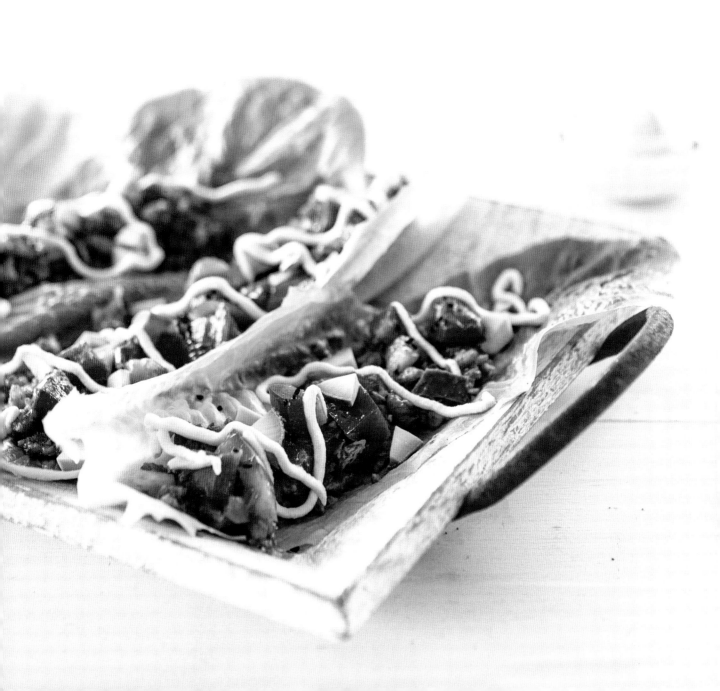

RAW PAD THAI WITH KELP NOODLES

NOODLES

1 zucchini, spiralised

1 cup shredded cabbage

½ packet kelp noodles (approx. 250g), washed and rinsed well

⅓ cup fresh coriander, finely chopped, with stalks

¼ cup sunflower or bean sprouts

1 red bell pepper, sliced thinly

2 spring onions, chopped

¾ cup raw activated cashew nuts, crushed

CREAMY THAI SAUCE

¼ cup almond butter

¼ cup tahini

¼ cup olive oil

1 tsp fresh ginger, grated

1 small clove of garlic

¼ cup fresh lime juice

2 tbs Coconut Magic coconut vinegar

2 tbs Coconut Magic coconut nectar

2 tbs tamari sauce

½ cup clean water, adding more if required for desired consistency

Noodles:

Place all the Noodle ingredients in a mixing bowl.

Creamy Thai Sauce:

Combine the Thai Sauce ingredients in a small blender and blend until smooth.

Pour the dressing over the mixture, coating the vegetables evenly.

Serve garnished with lime wedges, fresh coriander and spring onions.

Serves 4+ prep: 30 min.

Thai Sauce

This is an option for a stronger flavoured Thai Sauce.

¼ cup tamarind sauce
1 tbs Coconut Magic coconut nectar
1 tbs tamari sauce
Pinch of pink salt

Mix all ingredients together well and pour over the top of the noodle salad.

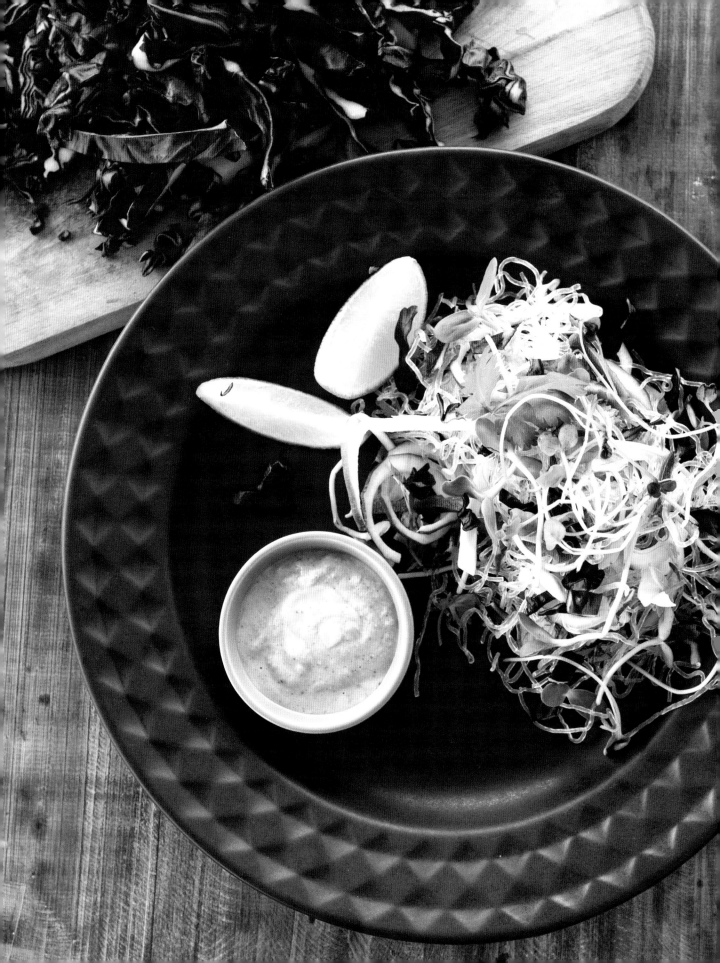

RAW VEGAN TUNA SALAD

1 cup sunflower seeds, soaked 2 hours

½ cup celery, chopped

½ cup shredded carrot

1 tbs Coconut Magic coconut vinegar

½ small red onion, finely chopped

½ tbs Coconut Magic coconut nectar

1 tbs fresh lemon juice

½ tsp herb salt

Freshly ground black pepper, to taste

½ cup cucumber, cut in slices to garnish

Paprika, to garnish

1 bunch of Romaine lettuce

Place all ingredients except paprika and cucumber in food processor. Pulse until just combined (you want to leave it a tiny bit chunky).

Remove from processor and stir in chopped cucumber.

Sprinkle with paprika and another small dusting of herb salt.

Serve in a lettuce leaf wrap with raw crackers.

Serves 4-6 + prep: 10 min + soaking time: 2 hr.

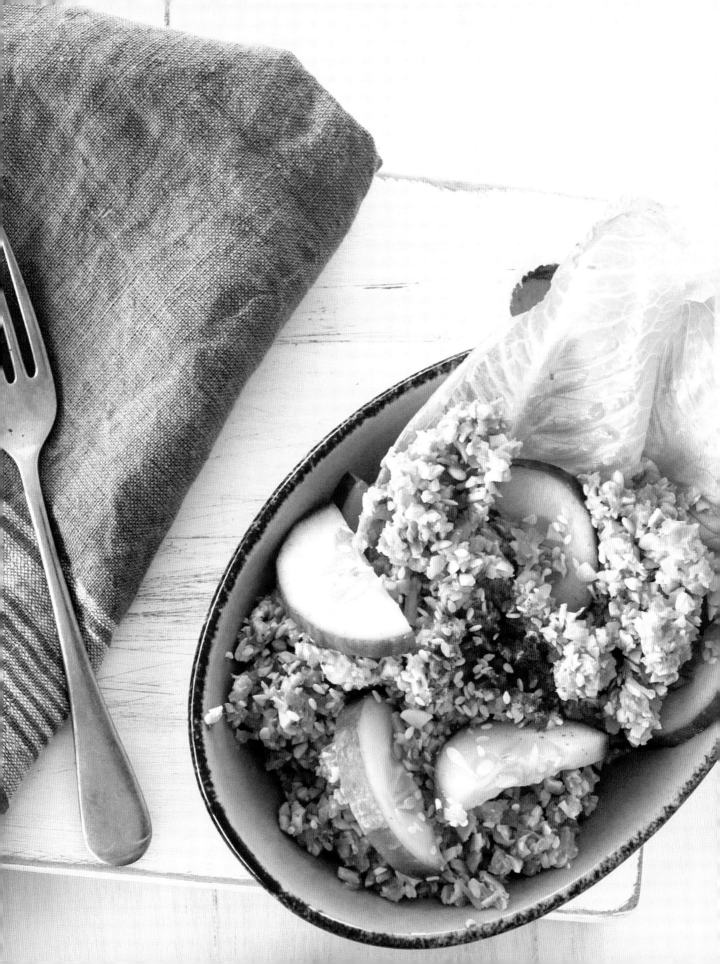

RAW VEGETABLE PATTIES

2 cups almonds

½ cup sunflower seeds

2 carrots, roughly chopped

1 zucchini, roughly chopped

½ cup dulse flakes

½ cup parsley

2 tbs Coconut Magic coconut oil

2 tbs olive oil

1 tbs cumin powder

1 tbs turmeric

1 tsp pink salt

In a food processor, process almonds, sunflower seeds, carrots and zucchini until well combined. The vegetables and seeds will become finely chopped and stick together.

Transfer to a large mixing bowl, combine all other ingredients and mix well.

Form into eleven 2¼ inch patties.

Dehydrate at 145 degrees for 2-3 hours or bake patties in the oven for 20 - 30 minutes, or until golden brown and warm.

Serve with Tahini Dressing sauce. (See page 182 for recipe).

Serves 4-6 + prep: 20 min. hr + dehydrate 2-3 hrs + cook: 20-30 min.

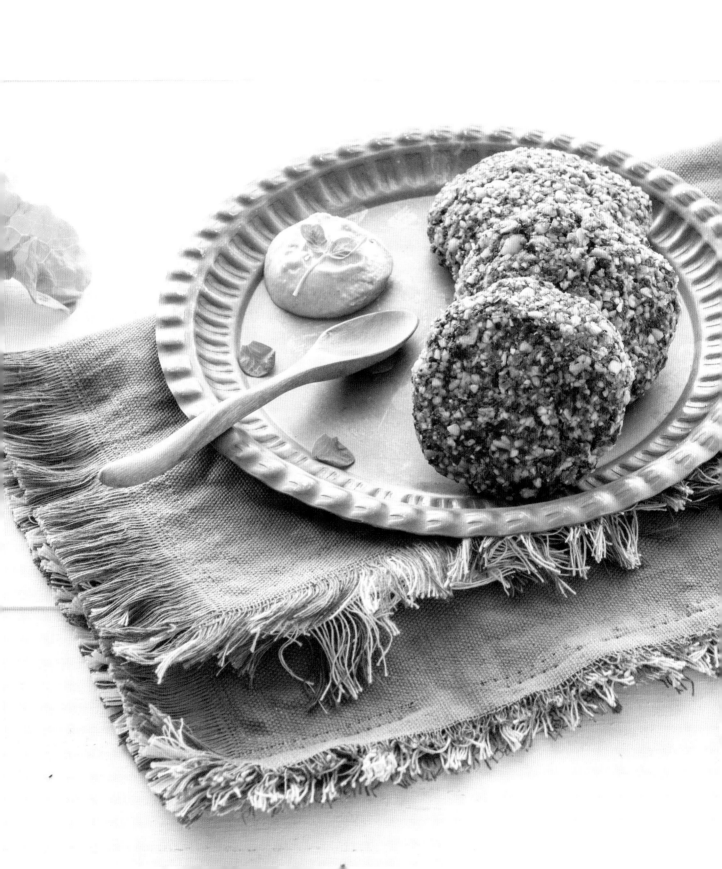

RAW LASAGNA

WALNUT BUTTER

1 cup walnuts

¼ cup red onion, chopped

Pinch of sea salt

5 tbs sundried tomatoes
(slice fresh tomatoes and
dehydrate for one day)

1 tsp paprika

½ cup shredded carrot

1 tbs olive oil

Pinch cayenne pepper

MACADAMIA CREAM

1 cup macadamia nuts

2 tbs lime juice

1 tbs red onion, chopped

1 tsp cumin powder

1 tsp pink salt

½ cup clean water
or coconut water

½ cup cashew nuts
(soaked for 2 hours)

Pinch cayenne pepper

2 tbs olive oil

PESTO PASTA

1 cup cashews (soaked 2 hours)

½ cup pine nuts

½ cup parsley

1 cup sweet basil leaf

¼ cup olive oil

1 tbs Italian seasoning

2 cloves garlic

½ tsp sea salt

TOMATO

1 red bell pepper

½ cup sundried tomato

1 tbs Coconut Magic
coconut vinegar

1 tbs miso paste

1 tsp Coconut Magic
coconut nectar

1 cup tomato, chopped

1 piece ginger

¼ cup pecan nuts

1 tsp turmeric

VEGETABLE SALAD

Zucchini – inside layers

Romaine lettuce – on the bottom

Cherry tomato – on top

Celery – inside

Walnut Butter: Blend in a food processor until creamy.

Macadamia Cream: Process all ingredients in a food processor until almost smooth.

Pesto Pasta: Process all ingredients in a food processor until smooth.

Tomato Butter: Process all ingredients in blender until smooth.

Vegetable Salad: Use a round cylinder to prepare the layers of the lasagne. Build the lasagna with equal layers of the sauces, one serve per plate on a bed of lettuce. Start with a layer of the walnut butter, cream cheese, zucchini, tomato sauce, celery, and pesto. Add another layer of zucchini to the top. Place the cylinder in the centre of the plate.

Remove the cylinder and the lasagna will stand alone.

Garnish with some cherry tomatoes and celery leaves.

This is best served immediately.
Serves 4 + prep: 60 – 70 min.

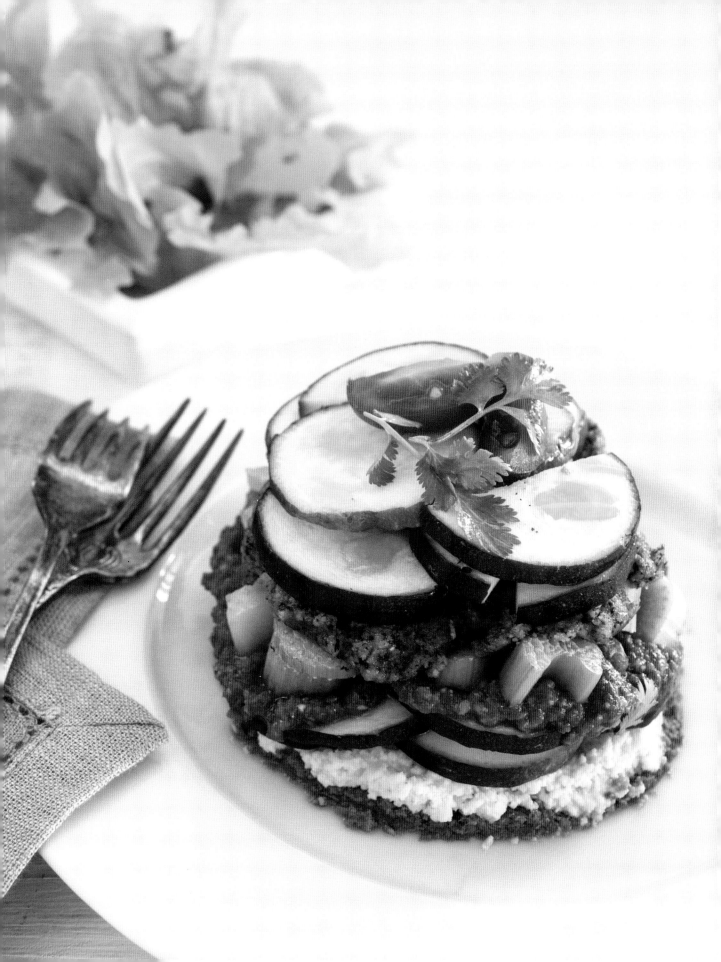

snacks, sides & dips

COCONUT AND CHIA HERBED CRACKERS

½ cup Coconut Magic coconut flour

¼ cup organic chia seed meal (grind chia seeds in a coffee grinder or blender. Store in a jar)

⅛ tsp pink salt

⅛ tsp garlic powder

½ tsp Italian seasoning

¼ cup Coconut Magic coconut oil

¾ cup hot water

Preheat the oven to 180°C (350°F). Using a whisk or fork, mix the dry ingredients in a bowl until well incorporated. Add in the coconut oil. Add the hot water a little at a time, stirring as you go. Mix well with a spoon, stirring and mashing out any lumps. Once the dough forms into a ball, place it on a baking-paper-lined tray and roll out. You can use parchment paper under your rolling pin to prevent sticking. Keep rolling your dough until it is as thin as you can get without tearing it. Slice into squares with a pizza cutter. Bake for approximately 20 to 25 minutes, or until crackers are crispy and brown.

Serves 6 + prep: 5 min. + cook: 10 min.

RAW HUMMUS

2 cups of chickpeas (soaked overnight)

1 clove garlic

1 tsp cumin powder

2 tbs tahini

¼ cup lemon juice

Pink salt, to taste

¼ cup olive oil

¼ cup Coconut Magic coconut oil, melted

Fresh parsley or coriander to garnish

2-4 tbs clean water to assist with blending

Blend all ingredients in a high-speed blender, adding water if required or until smooth and creamy. Use the tamp attachment to keep it all moving. Serve with chopped carrot, celery and or crackers.

Makes 15 small serves + prep: 15 min. soaking: overnight

ZUCCHINI DIP

1 cup sunflower seeds, soaked for 2 hours then drained

2 small cloves garlic

2 tbs lemon juice

Pink salt (to taste)

¼ cup olive oil

¼ cup Coconut Magic coconut oil, melted

3 medium zucchini cut into 1 inch (2½ cm) pieces

¼ cup fresh parsley

Grind the sunflower seeds in a food processor until they are creamy. Set the paste aside in a bowl.

Blend all other ingredients in a blender until almost pureed. Use the tamp attachment to keep it all moving. Add the sunflower paste to the blender and blend together. Serve with chopped carrot, celery and or crackers.

Serves 6 + prep: 5 min. + cook: 10 min

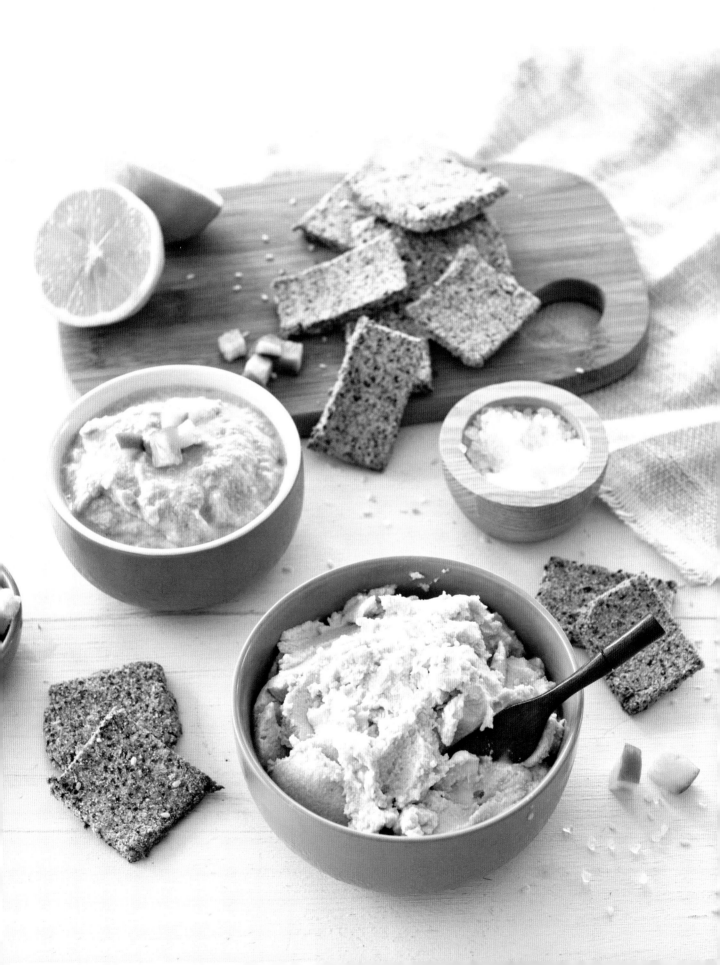

SALT & VINEGAR KALE CHIPS

½ cup sunflower seeds

2 tbs olive oil

1 tbs Coconut Magic
coconut vinegar

½ tbs balsamic vinegar

1 tsp pink salt (to taste)

1 large bunch curly kale -
wash and strip the kale leaves
discarding the stems.

Combine the vinegars and olive oil, sunflower seeds and salt in a food processor. Pulse until a chunky paste is created, add a little water if required to assist with the process.

Put the kale leaves in a bowl. Pour the mixture from the food processor over the top of the kale leaves, and using clean hands massage the mixture into the kale, to evenly coat the leaves.

Using the Dehydrator:

Warm the dehydrator to 46°C (115°F).

Spread the kale leaves out onto 4 mesh trays.

Dehydrate for approximately 12 hours or until the kale becomes crispy.

Using the Oven:

Pre-heat the oven to 95°C (200° F).

Line a baking tray with parchment paper. Spread the kale on top of the baking sheet, as evenly as you can. Bake for about 2 hours. The time may vary so keep an eye on the kale to make sure it doesn't burn. When it's dried out and crispy, it's ready to eat.

Enjoy immediately or keep in an airtight container for 2 weeks.

Serves 6-8 + prep: 20 min. + cook: 2 hours or dehydrating: 12 hr.

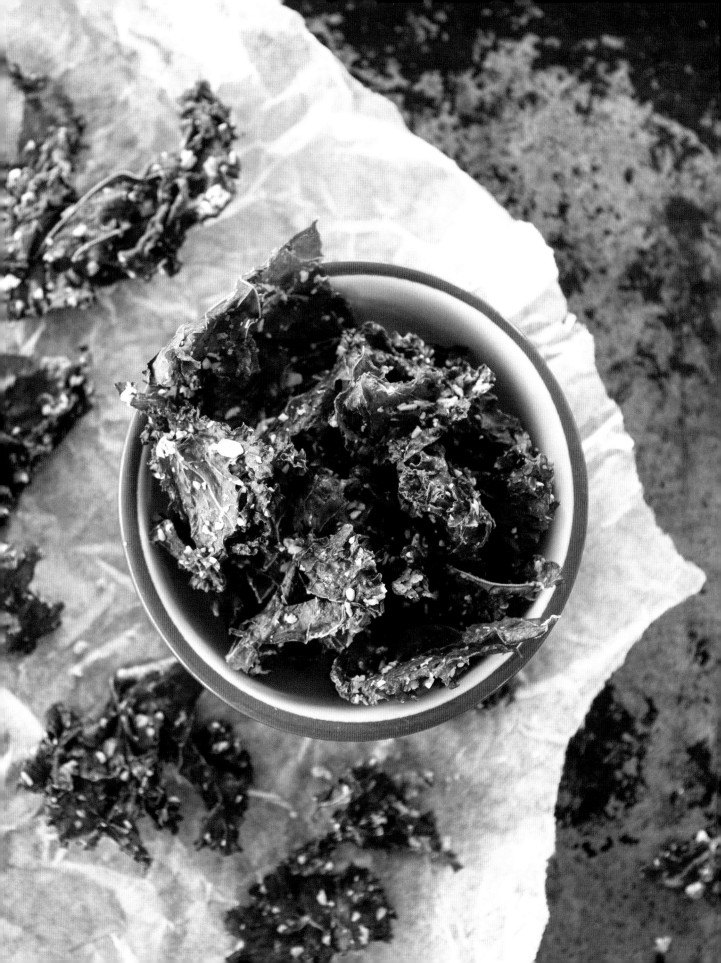

CHEESY BROCCOLI

_____

2 tbs nutritional yeast

½ tsp sweet paprika

¼ tsp garlic powder

¼ cup tahini

1 tsp Coconut Magic coconut nectar

2 tbs Coconut Magic coconut oil, melted

3 tbs clean water

1 tbs Coconut Magic coconut vinegar

⅓ cup Coconut Magic coconut flakes, toasted

1 large head of broccoli, broken up into small florets

In a small mixing bowl combine the nutritional yeast, sweet paprika and garlic powder. Stir in the tahini and mix well. Pour in the coconut oil, coconut nectar, water and coconut vinegar. Whisk all ingredients together well. If you prefer a thinner sauce add some more water. Place the broccoli florets into a large bowl. Pour the sauce over the top until the broccoli is well coated, use your hands if required to ensure the broccoli is well covered. Put 1 tbs of coconut oil in a pan over a medium heat, place the coconut flakes in the pan for just 1-2 minutes, or until golden brown. Sprinkle the toasted coconut flakes over the cheesy broccoli and serve immediately.

Serves 4-6 + prep: 20 min.

BLANCHED ASPARAGUS WITH FLAX-OIL DRESSING

_____

1 bunch of organic asparagus. (Remove the woody ends from the asparagus by gently bending the end of each spear until it snaps naturally)

3 cups clean water

3 tbs flaxseed oil

2 tbs hemp seeds

Pink salt, to taste

Bring a pan of water to the boil. (Ideally the whole asparagus spear should fit inside the pan.) Add the asparagus and cook for 2 minutes or until bright green.

Run under cold water to stop the cooking process.

Dress with salt and flaxseed oil.

Sprinkle with nutritional yeast if desired for a cheesy flavor. Or with hemp seeds for added protein. Serve immediately.

Serves 4-6 + prep: 20 min.

ROASTED CAULIFLOWER WITH COCONUT + SPICE

_____

2 tsp garam masala

1 tsp curry powder (optional)

2 tsp pink salt, to taste

6 tbs Coconut Magic coconut oil, melted

1 head cauliflower – stem removed, cut into medium florets

Preheat the oven to 200°C (390°F).

In a small mixing bowl combine coconut oil, the spices and the salt. Toss the cauliflower through this mix until it's thoroughly covered in coconut oil and spices.

Line an oven tray with baking paper. Transfer the cauliflower to the tray and roast in the oven (stirring halfway) until the cauliflower is caramelised around the edges. When it's crisp and tender, it's ready to eat. Serve hot straight from the oven.

Serves 4-6 + prep: 20 min. + cook: 15-20 min.

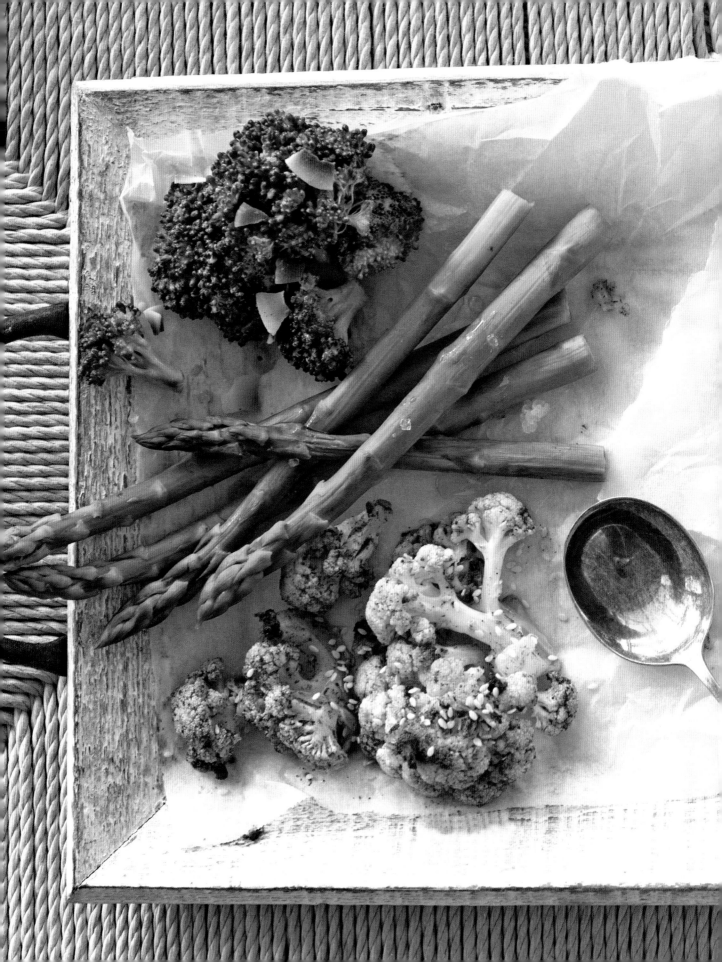

TOMATO SAUCE

8 tomatoes

1 tbs basil leaves

2 tbs red onion

½ tsp pink salt

1 tbs Coconut Magic coconut vinegar

1 Medjool date

Pink salt and pepper, to taste

Blend ingredients all together in a blender until well combined. You can add some Italian herbs for an Italian flavour.

Serves 8-10 + prep: 15 min.

AVOCADO SALSA

2 large ripe avocados

2 tbs olive oil

1 tbs Coconut Magic coconut oil (optional)

1 tomato or ½ red capsicum, chopped into small square pieces

1 spring onion, washed and finely sliced

2-3 tbs lemon juice, to taste

½ tsp pink salt, to taste

1-2 tbs fresh coriander, chopped

Pinch cayenne pepper (optional)

Mash the avocado flesh together with the olive and coconut oils until it all becomes soft and creamy. Don't worry if you have a few lumps –it adds to the salsa texture.

Add chopped capsicum/ tomato, spring onion, lemon, salt, pepper (if using) and coriander and mix all ingredients together well.

Serves 8-10 + prep: 15 min.

COCONUT CRUSTED SWEET POTATO CHIPS

1 large sweet potato, sliced into thin-shaped chips

¼ cup Coconut Magic coconut flour

¼ cup Coconut Magic desiccated coconut

½ cup Coconut Magic coconut oil, melted

1 tsp pink salt, to taste

1 tsp pepper, to taste

1 tsp cinnamon powder

Parsley to garnish

2 tbs Coconut Magic coconut vinegar (optional for salt and vinegar flavoured chips)

Preheat the oven to 180°C (350° F).

Mix the coconut flour and the desiccated coconut together in a bowl. Add salt, pepper and cinnamon to taste. Place the powder mixture inside a zip lock bag. Use a silicone brush, or your hands, to cover the sweet potato chips in coconut oil.

Place a few chips at a time inside the zip lock bag and shake them around until the powder has evenly and lightly coated the potatoes. Coat a baking tray with some coconut oil. Lay the chips evenly on the tray and place the tray in the oven.

Bake the chips in the oven for 20 minutes, flip them over and bake for another 15-20 minutes or until nicely crusted and brown.

Sprinkle parsley on top and enjoy with some coconut vinegar (optional), and some tomato sauce or avocado salsa. Serve immediately.

Serves 4 + prep: 20 min. + cook: 35-40 min.

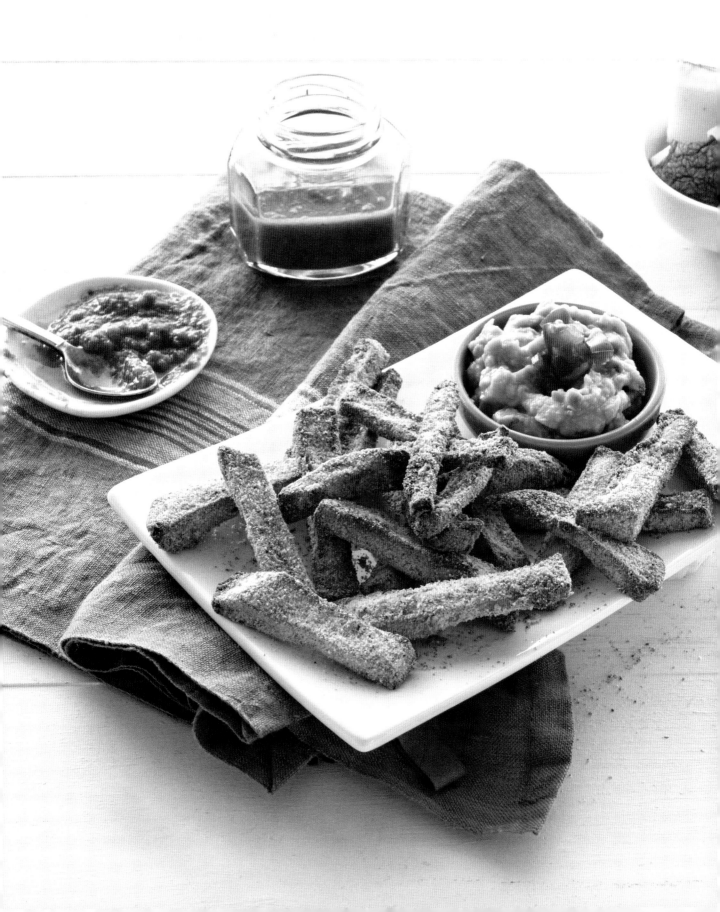

super salads &
salad dressings

KALE & AVOCADO
SALAD WITH SWEET MISO

─────────────────────

KALE SALAD

1 large bunch of kale, washed well,
stems removed

1 tbs olive oil

1 cucumber, peeled and diced

1 large avocado, diced

1 small red onion, diced

¼ cup pine nuts

1 red capsicum, chopped into
very small pieces

10 cherry tomatoes, chopped in half

SWEET MISO DRESSING

1 tbs white miso paste

1 tbs Coconut Magic coconut nectar

¼ cup Coconut Magic coconut vinegar

¼ cup olive oil

1 tbs minced fresh ginger

Salad:

Chop kale into small pieces, place into a bowl and pour olive oil over the leaves. Massage oil into the kale to soften. Add all other salad ingredients to the bowl. Mix well.

Sweet Miso Dressing:

In a glass jar, combine the miso, coconut nectar and vinegar and mix well. Add the oil and ginger and shake well. (You can also let it sit for 24 hours, or at least overnight, to allow the ginger to mellow and infuse.)

Blend all ingredients together in a blender until well mixed. Add the sweet miso dressing to the salad and mix well.

Serves 2-4 as a salad meal + prep: 20 min.

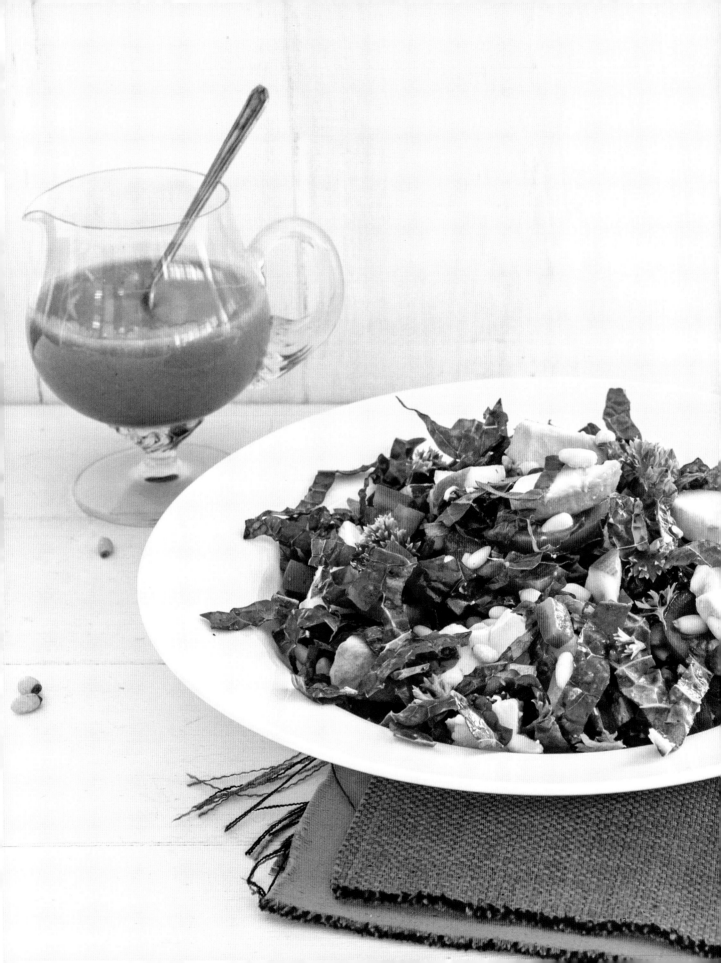

GREEK SALAD WITH ALMOND FETA

SALAD

Large bowl of lettuce leaves, washed

1 cup cherry tomatoes

1 small red onion, sliced

1 Lebanese cucumber

1 green capsicum, chopped

½ cup pitted black olives

1 red capsicum, chopped

½ cup fresh mint leaves, finely chopped

DRESSING

½ cup olive oil

¼ cup Coconut Magic coconut vinegar

2 tsp dried oregano

Pinch of pink salt

ALMOND FETA

1½ cups almond meal

¼ cup lemon juice

3 tbs olive oil

1 clove crushed garlic

½ tsp pink salt

Salad:

Wash the greens and vegetables well, then shake or pat dry with a tea towel.

Using your hands, break up the green leaves into small pieces and place into a bowl.

Add all other salad ingredients and mix well, using your hands.

Dressing:

Blend all ingredients and pour into a small jar.

Almond Feta:

Preheat oven to 180°C (350°F)

Process all ingredients in food processor until a smooth paste consistency is reached (approximately 4-6 minutes).

Turn mixture out onto a sheet of plastic wrap, and use the plastic wrap to shape it into a tight disc about 3 cm (1.25 inch) thick.

Bake on a baking sheet lined with parchment paper for 15-25 minutes, until the surface is crusty and slightly golden. Let cool.

Add sliced almond feta to the salad.

Serves 4 + prep: 15 min. cook: 15-25 min.

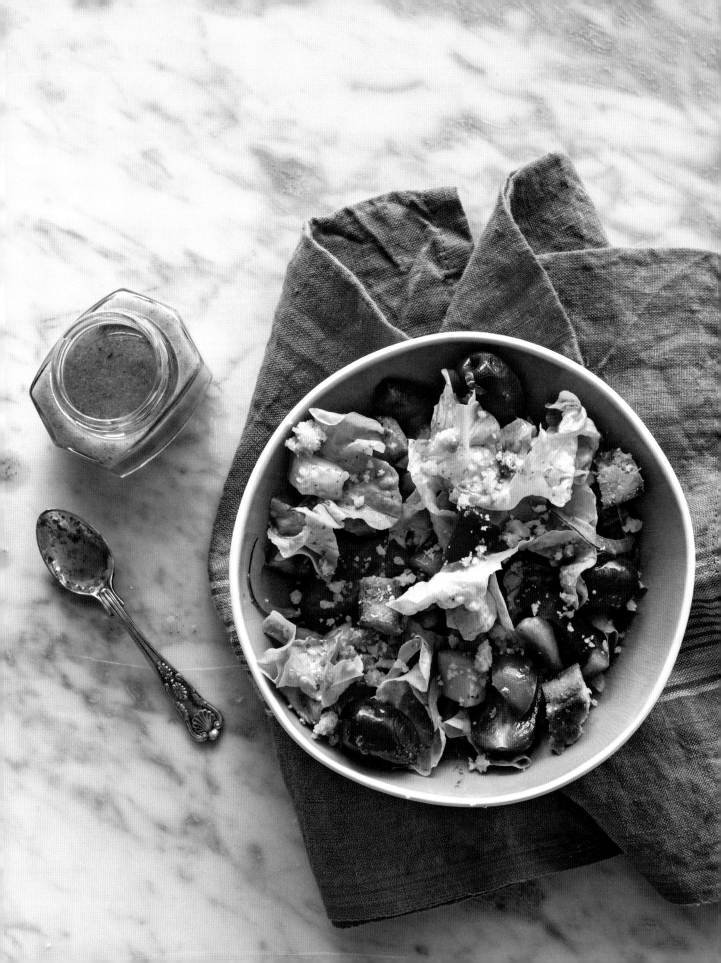

QUINOA HERB SALAD

QUINOA SALAD

1 cup quinoa, washed and drained

2 cups clean water

1 handful curly parsley, washed and chopped

1 bunch fresh coriander, washed and chopped

1 red capsicum, chopped

1 green capsicum, chopped

1 red onion, diced

6-7 fresh mint leaves, chopped

THE DRESSING

½ cup extra virgin olive oil

3 tbs Coconut Magic coconut vinegar

1 tsp lemon juice

½ tsp each thyme, basil and oregano

1 small clove of garlic

1 tsp pink salt, to taste

Quinoa Salad:

Wash the quinoa well using clean water and a strainer. This washes away the bitter saponins on the surface of the seeds.

Add the quinoa to a medium-sized pot with 2 cups of water, bring the mixture to a boil.

Cover and simmer for approximately 15 minutes, or until the water is fully absorbed. Remove from heat and stir the quinoa so it separates and becomes fluffy.

Leave the quinoa to cool then add all other salad ingredients.

The Dressing:

Blend all ingredients and pour into a small jar.

Add the dressing to Quinoa salad and mix together well.

The salad will become crisp, fresh and tasty, as the flavours of the dressing blend in with the vegetables and quinoa.

Serves 4 as a salad meal + prep: 15 min. cooking: 15 min.

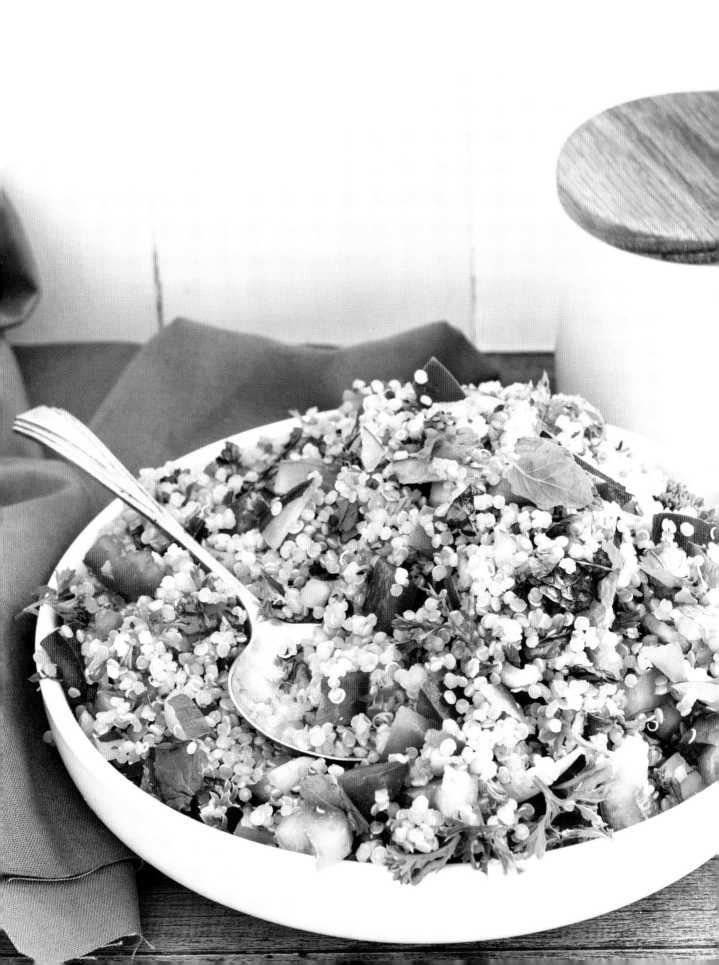

SPICY LENTIL SALAD

SALAD

½ red onion, finely chopped

1 small clove garlic, minced (optional)

10 cherry tomatoes, cut in half

2 tsp lemon juice

¼ cup coriander, chopped

2 tbs fresh basil leaves, chopped

1 cup lentils

1 green capsicum, chopped into small pieces

THE SPICY DRESSING

2 tsp Coconut Magic coconut vinegar

2 tsp olive oil

1 tsp ground coriander powder

¼ tsp pink salt, to taste

¼ tsp fresh cayenne pepper (optional for the added spice)

For Sprouted Lentils:

Place the lentils in a glass bowl, cover with two cups of clean water. Cover with a gauze or cloth, and seal with a rubber band. Soak no less than 15 hours.

Drain, rinse and turn the jar upside down to clean the bottom layer. This prevents rotting.

Rinse with pure clean water twice per day, even when germination begins.

Sprouting usually starts to occur from four to five days. It is well worth the wait to enjoy this delicious and nutritious crunchy texture.

For Cooked Lentils:

Place the lentils in a bowl and soak for a minimum of 2 hours. Overnight works best.

Put 2 cups of water in a saucepan and bring to the boil.

Add the lentils and cook for about 30 minutes, or until soft.

Rinse well with cool filtered water to reduce the temperature of the cooked lentils.

Salad:

Place onions, garlic, tomatoes and lemon juice into a medium bowl and mix well.

Add the remainder of the ingredients and mix. Add salt to taste.

Serve in bowls. This is great as a side dish with some raw soup.

Serves 4 as a side meal or 2 as a meal + prep: 25 min.

Take note...

Only use organic seeds, legumes, grains and nuts for sprouting. Non-organic produce contains chemicals and may not sprout.

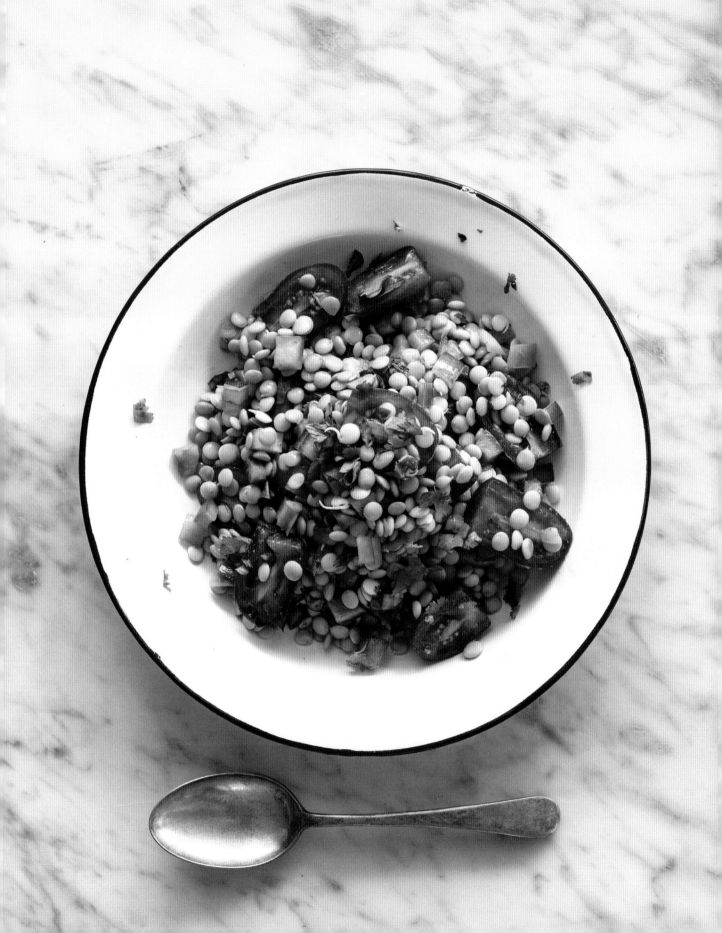

STEAMED GREEN VEGETABLE SALAD

VEGETABLE SALAD

1 head of broccoli

½ cup snow peas, stems removed

1 zucchini, sliced

1 bunch asparagus, chopped in half

1 cup green beans, chopped in half

3 pieces squash, chopped into quarters

1 cup fresh spinach leaves, washed and drained

½ cup sunflower sprouts

2 tbs fresh basil leaves, chopped

2 tbs pumpkin seeds, to garnish

DRESSING

½ cup flaxseed oil

¼ cup lemon juice, to taste

Pink salt, to taste

Vegetable Salad:

Steam the broccoli, snow peas, zucchini, asparagus, beans and squash for 5- 10 minutes on low heat. Don't let the vegetables get too soft.

Rinse under cold water to bring back to room temperature. Drain well.

In a large bowl, mix the steamed ingredients together with the spinach, sunflower sprouts and basil leaves.

Dressing:

Add flaxseed oil, lemon and salt to taste.

Garnish with pumpkin seeds.

Serves 4 as a side dish or 2 as a meal + prep: 25 min.

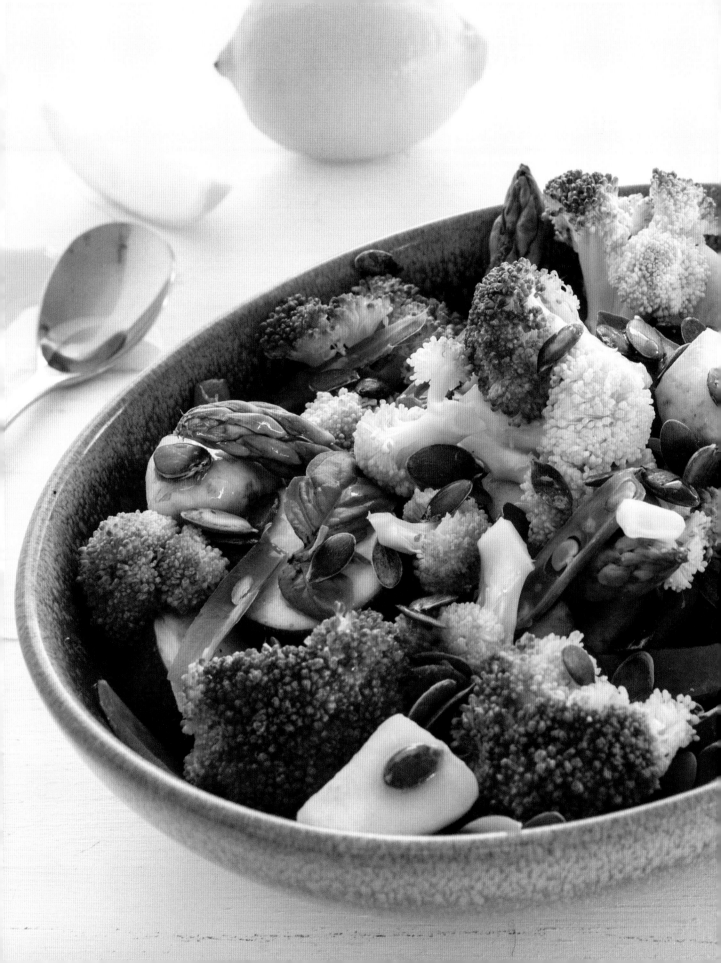

COLESLAW + COCONUT CITRUS VINAIGRETTE

COLESLAW

2 cups green cabbage, shredded

½ cup red cabbage, shredded

1½ cups carrots, julienned

1 small red onion, shredded

Pink salt and pepper, to taste

I handful parsley, chopped finely

White sesame seeds and orange slices to garnish

COCONUT CITRUS VINAIGRETTE

2 tbs Coconut Magic coconut vinegar

½ tsp pink salt, to taste

¼ tsp black pepper, to taste

¼ cup fresh orange juice

1 tbs mustard

1 small clove garlic

¼ cup Coconut Magic coconut oil (melted)

¼ cup extra virgin olive oil

Coleslaw :

In a large mixing bowl, add red and green cabbage, carrots, red onion and parsley.

Dressing:

Combine all ingredients except the oils and mix well.

Drizzle in the oils slowly, and continue mixing.

Add the dressing to the coleslaw, and mix to combine.

Add salt and fresh cracked pepper to taste.

Serve at room temperature or chilled. This is a great salad to make ahead of time covered an hour or so on the counter or in the fridge for longer.

Serve with a sprinkle of white sesame seeds over the top and slices of orange.

Serves 6 as a side meal or 3 as a meal + prep: 25 min.

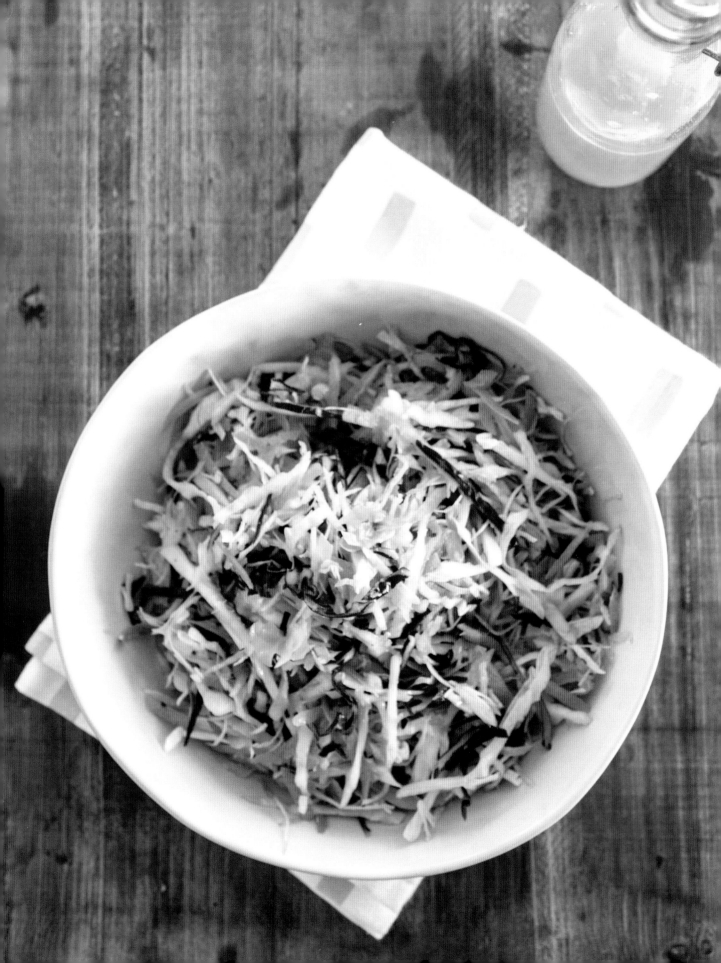

HEMPSEED TABOULI

3 cups fresh parsley, washed and drained

1 cup fresh mint leaves, washed and drained

¼ tsp pink salt, to taste

1 tomato, chopped into very small pieces

1 cup hemp seeds

1 small red onion, chopped finely

2 tbs olive oil

2 tbs lemon juice

Process the parsley, mint and salt in a food processor until minced.

Transfer to a large mixing bowl.

Add the tomatoes, hemp seeds, onion, oil and lemon juice. Mix all ingredients together well.

Serve in bowls. This is great as a side dish with falafels or with some raw burgers.

Serves 4 + prep: 15 min.

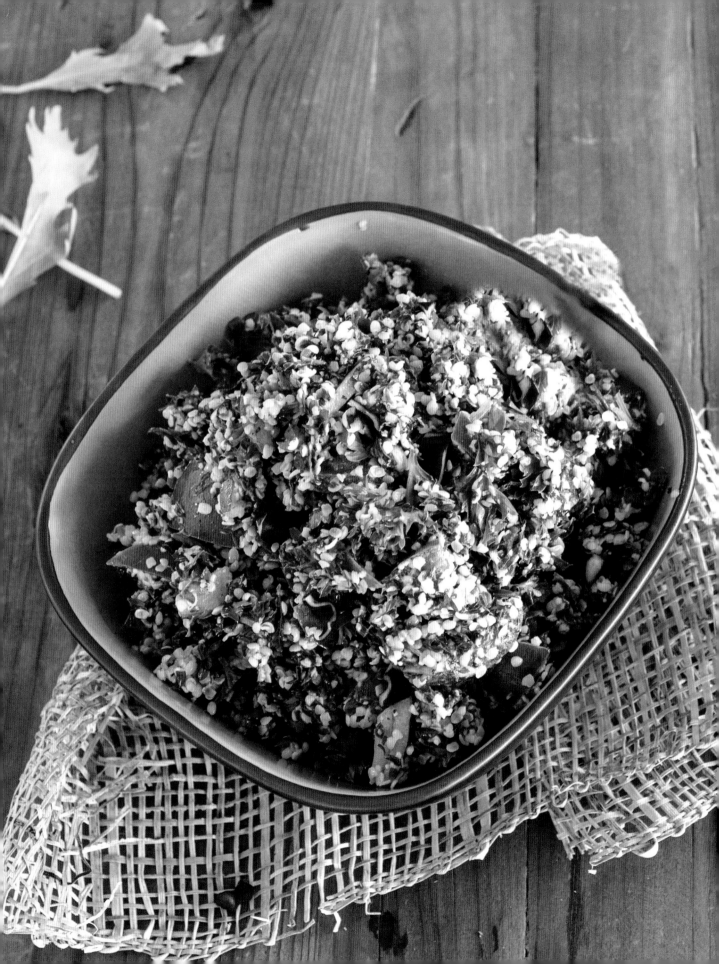

CREAMY CORIANDER

½ ripe avocado

¾ cup packed fresh coriander

½ cup plain coconut yoghurt

2 scallions, chopped

1 clove garlic, quartered

1 tbs lime juice

½ tsp Coconut Magic coconut sugar

½ tsp pink salt

Place all ingredients in a blender; blend until smooth.

Serves to taste + prep: 5 min.

TAHINI DRESSING

¼ cup lemon juice

1 ½ cups olive oil

⅓ cup tahini

1 tbs Coconut Magic coconut nectar

1 small clove garlic, minced

1 tsp pink salt

Freshly ground pepper, to taste

Combine lemon juice, olive oil, tahini, coconut nectar and garlic in a blender, a jar with a tight-fitting lid or a medium bowl.

Blend, shake or whisk until smooth. Season with salt and pepper.

Optional: Add ¼ cup each basil and parsley leaves, and 2 tbs pine nuts for a creamy tahini herbed dressing.

Serves to taste + prep: 5 min.

AVOCADO AIOLI DRESSING

1 large whole avocado

1 small garlic clove

¼ cup lemon juice

1 tsp Coconut Magic coconut nectar

2 tbs basil leaves

¼ small red onion, chopped

½ tsp pink salt, to taste

¼ cup olive oil

Blend ingredients in the blender until smooth and creamy.

NB. Add an additional whole avocado, 1 tbs of basil leaves, and 1 tbs of lemon juice, for a thicker aioli dip consistency.

Serves to taste + prep: 5 min.

BASIC VINAIGRETTE

¼ cup olive oil

2 tbs Coconut Magic coconut vinegar

Pink salt and pepper, to taste

Mix all ingredients together in a bowl or blend all ingredients together in a mini blender. Add ½ teaspoon Italian herbs and ½ teaspoon minced garlic for Italian vinaigrette.

Serves to taste + prep: 5 min.

Take note...

Salad dressings will last up to 5 days in a sealed jar in the fridge.

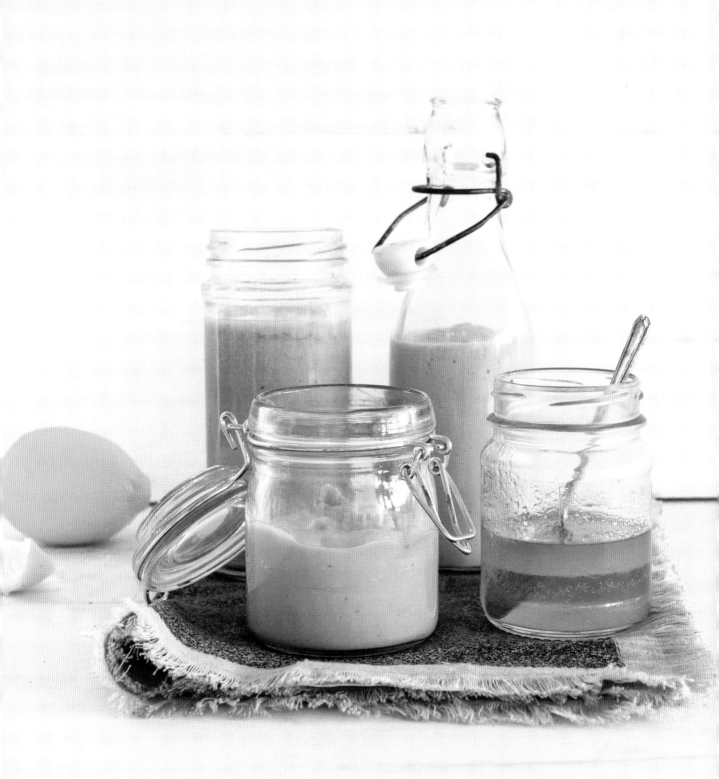

raw chocolate

INTRODUCTION TO RAW CHOCOLATE

The simple pleasure of eating raw chocolate can keep you healthy and give you an abundance of energy.

As coconut is known as the Queen of Mother Nature, cacao is known as the King. When you combine the two you create a power force of love and nutrition.

Chocolate is something that appeals to the emotions and the taste buds.

In the past, I felt guilty about eating chocolate. I thought it was unhealthy and fattening, as well as damaging to the environment while being harvested. It wasn't always a food of choice for me – more like an addictive fix.

But don't head off to Chocoholics Anonymous just yet!

Chocolate, when eaten in its raw unaltered state, is not only delicious but good for you! Of course, this is not the sugar-laden commercial chocolate variety, which is over-heated and filled with chemicals to give it a long shelf-life and prevent it from melting in warmer temperatures. This is real, raw chocolate. Once you taste it, you will never want to go back to mainstream commercial chocolate.

There is something about eating chocolate that lifts the spirits and satisfies the body. Just like coconut, pure cacao is grown in the tropics, and it was prized by the ancients. The Aztecs and Mayans ground cacao into a spiced drink that was consumed during their ceremonies and rituals.

Raw cacao has not been heat-treated, so all of its nutrients remain intact. When combined with health-giving ingredients such as coconut oil, desiccated coconut, coconut nectar, pink salt, fresh berries, cinnamon and maca powder, it makes a healthy, tasty treat.

Some of the great things you will find in raw chocolate include: Magnesium, iron, copper, calcium, serotonin, tryptophan, phenylethylamine (pea), polyphenols, histamine, epicatechins, dopamine, tyramine and salsolinol.

So, now you can make your own raw chocolate.

Pour it over fruits, blend it into a mousse, spice it up in your hot cacao drink, and combine it with your favourite superfoods.

RAW CACAO & COCONUT FUDGE

This sweet treat is made from a rich and creamy blend of raw anti-oxidant rich cacao, slimming coconut oil, a creamy base of blended cashews and pure nutrient-rich, low GI coconut nectar - with an added crunch of cacao nibs. These cacao fudge babies are kept raw to maintain maximum superfood nutrients.

1 cup raw cashews, soaked for 1-2 hours

½ cup raw cacao powder

¼ cup Coconut Magic coconut nectar

¼ cup Coconut Magic coconut oil

1 tsp pure vanilla extract

¼ cup raw cacao nibs

2 tbs Coconut Magic desiccated coconut

Pinch of pink salt

Drain and rinse the cashews. Place the cashews, coconut oil, coconut nectar, vanilla, cacao powder and pink salt into a food processor and pulse until smooth and creamy. Stop every now and then to scrape the sides of the bowl.

Transfer the mixture into a medium-size bowl and stir in the cacao nibs until they are well combined and evenly distributed.

Place a piece of waxed baking paper on a flat plate. Spread the fudge evenly. Using a knife make rectangle-shaped pieces of fudge from the mixture. Place each piece on top of the baking paper tray until all of the mixture has been used up.

Sprinkle desiccated coconut over the top of the fudge pieces. Place another piece of baking paper carefully over the top of the fudge pieces. Freeze until solid, 3-4 hours.

Remove from the freezer and lift the frozen fudge from the tray using the waxed paper.

Makes 15 pieces + prep: 20 min. cooling: 3 – 4 hr. soaking: 1 – 2 hr.

BERRY COCONUT CHOCOLATE

½ cup Coconut Magic coconut oil, melted

¼ cup cacao butter

½ cup cacao powder

¼ cup Coconut Magic coconut flakes

2 tbs Coconut Magic coconut nectar

2 tbs Coconut Magic coconut sugar,

1 cup mixed berries (blueberries, cherries, raspberries), washed and drained

1 tsp vanilla extract

Pinch of pink salt

Place the cacao butter in a small saucepan and place this saucepan inside a larger saucepan filled with boiling water, to melt. Add the coconut oil if this needs melting also. Add all other ingredients and mix well.

Place in a tray lined with baking paper, and place in the freezer for 2-4 hours to set. Remove from the freezer, break up into small pieces and your chocolate is ready to enjoy.

Serves 4 -6 + prep: 20 min. + cooling: 2-4 hours

WHITE CHOCOLATE

½ cup cacao butter, melted

½ cup coconut butter, melted

½ cup Coconut Magic coconut oil, melted

1 tsp vanilla powder

¼ cup Coconut Magic coconut nectar

½ cup cashews, soaked for 4 hours

Pinch of pink salt

1 drop lemon essential oil (optional)

Blend all ingredients together in a blender. Pour into chocolate moulds. Set in the freezer for 2-4 hours.

Makes 15 pieces + prep: 20 min. cooling: 2 -4 hr. soaking: 4 hr.

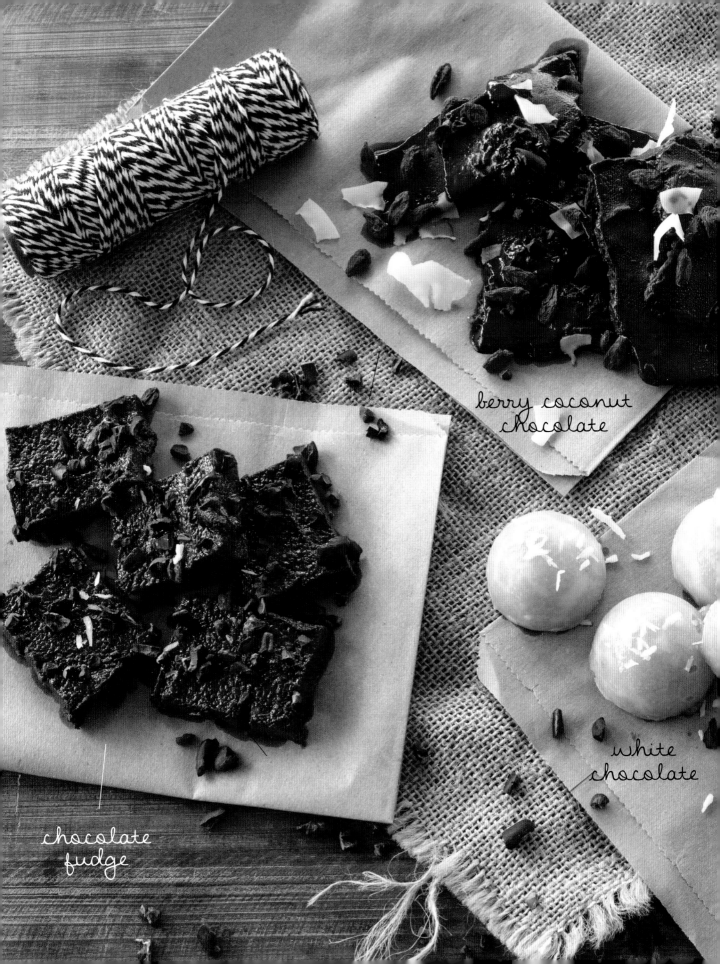

berry coconut
chocolate

white
chocolate

chocolate
fudge

BOUNTY BARS

FILLING

3 tbs cashews, soaked for a few hours and rinsed well

3 cups Coconut Magic shredded coconut

2 tbs Coconut Magic coconut flour

¼ cup Coconut Magic coconut oil, melted

¼ cup Coconut Magic coconut nectar

½ tsp vanilla powder

Pinch of pink salt

CHOCOLATE COATING

½ cup melted Coconut Magic coconut oil

½ cup cacao butter

½ cup cacao powder

¼ Coconut Magic coconut nectar

½ tsp vanilla powder

Pinch of pink salt

In a food processor, process all the ingredients for the filling. Pulse until a soft-crumbled and sticky texture is formed. Allow the filling to rest in the freezer for 15 minutes.

For the chocolate coating, melt the cacao butter and the coconut oil in a saucepan.

Blend all the chocolate coating ingredients together in a blender.

Remove the filling from the freezer and, with your hands, shape into rectangle bounty bars. (See image on opposite page).

Using a fork, dip each ball into the chocolate sauce, coating as thoroughly as you can.

Place each coated ball on a non-stick sheet or sheet of grease-proof paper.

Place in the fridge until the chocolate has set. Enjoy straight from the fridge or freezer.

Serves 15 pieces + prep: 30 min.
cooling: 2 hr. soaking: 2 – 3 hr.

MACA MACAROONS

MACA BALL

½ cup almonds, soaked for 4 hours

1 tbs maca powder

¼ cup cacao powder

½ tsp vanilla essence

2 tbs flax seed, ground

1 ¾ cups Coconut Magic desiccated coconut

5 pitted Medjool dates

2 tbs Coconut Magic coconut nectar

Pinch of pink salt

Coconut Magic desiccated coconut to garnish

Process all the ingredients except the desiccated coconut in a food processor and pulse until it becomes like a sticky dough.

Add one cup of the desiccated coconut and pulse until it is almost fully mixed through.

If the macaroon dough is not sticky enough, add some water and continue to pulse.

Transfer the mixture from the processor into a bowl and add the rest of the desiccated coconut. Mix it in well.

Form the mixture into 15 mini macaroon shapes and coat lightly with some more desiccated coconut.

Place in the fridge for 1-2 hours to set.

Makes 12 Maca Macaroons + prep: 15 min.
cooling: 1 – 2 hr.

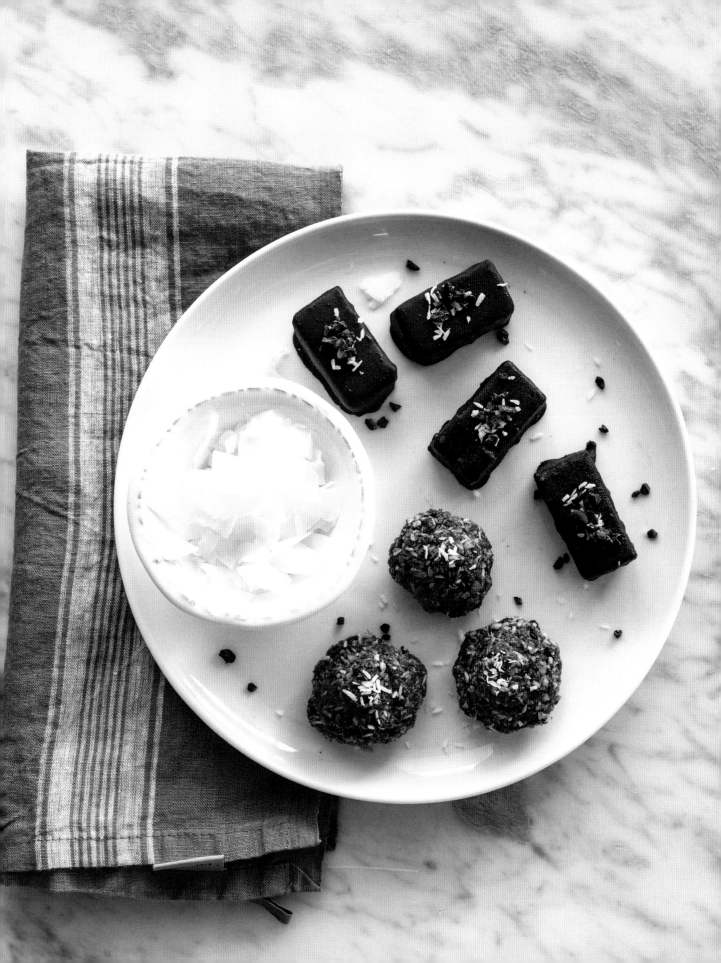

COCONUT PEPPERMINT SLICE

FIRST LAYER

¾ cup raw almond butter

¼ cup Coconut Magic coconut oil, melted

⅓ cup cacao powder

⅓ cup Coconut Magic coconut sugar

¼ tsp vanilla essence

Pinch of pink salt

SECOND LAYER

2 cups Coconut Magic desiccated coconut

⅔ cup coconut butter, softened

3 tbs Coconut Magic coconut nectar

1-2 tsp organic vanilla essence

THIRD LAYER: PEPPERMINT CHOCOLATE SAUCE

½ cup cacao powder

¼ cup Coconut Magic coconut nectar

½ cup Coconut Magic coconut oil, melted

Pinch of pink salt

½ tsp vanilla essence

1 drop peppermint essential oil

First layer:

Process all ingredients from the first layer in a food processor until well combined.

Pour into an oiled, parchment-lined 8 x 8-inch glass pan.

Set aside in refrigerator. This layer should be firm but not completely hard before adding the next layer.

Second layer:

Put the desiccated coconut in a medium-sized bowl. In a separate bowl whisk together the coconut butter, coconut nectar and vanilla essence. Pour over the desiccated coconut and mix well.

Put this layer over the first layer, gently patting down, and refrigerate to set.

Third Layer: Peppermint Chocolate Sauce:

Whisk together all ingredients for Peppermint Chocolate Sauce in a food processor.

Place this on top of the second layer, making sure to cover the whole layer.

Refrigerate for 2 or more hours before slicing and serving.

Serves 8 + prep: 30 min. cooling: at least 2 hours

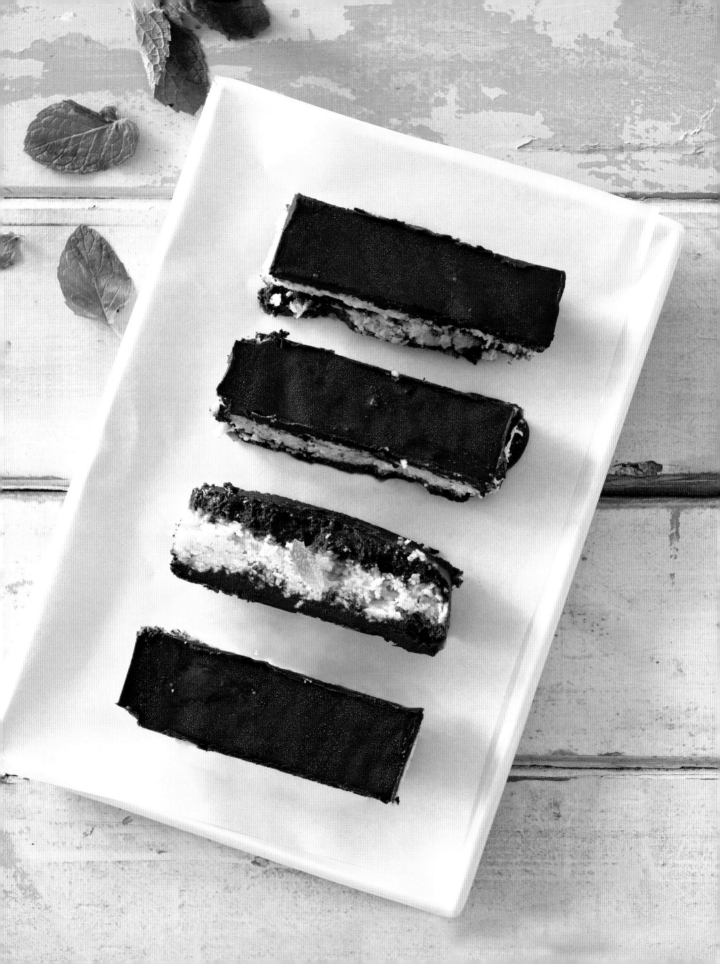

CHOCOLATE MOUSSE

MOUSSE

3 ripe avocados

½ cup raw cashews

½ cup Coconut Magic coconut oil

½ cup cacao powder

½ cup Coconut Magic coconut nectar

¼ tsp cinnamon powder

1 tsp vanilla essence

Pinch of pink salt

Cacao nibs to garnish

TOASTED COCONUT FLAKES

1-2 tbs Coconut Magic coconut oil

½ cup Coconut Magic coconut flakes

Chocolate Mousse:

Add all ingredients to the blender. Start at a low speed and gradually increase until all ingredients have become smooth and creamy. Use the tamper to assist and add a little water if required to achieve the desired consistency.

Refrigerate for 2 hours before serving. This will create a light and fluffy chocolate mousse consistency.

Toasted Coconut Flakes:

Add the coconut oil to the saucepan over a medium heat. Add the coconut flakes and toss for 1-2 minutes, or until golden brown. Allow the coconut flakes to cool before serving.

Serve the chocolate mousse with cacao nibs and toasted coconut flakes on top.

serves 4 - 6 + prep: 15 min. cooling: 2 hr.

Notes

You can also replace the avocado with fresh or frozen coconut meat for a delicious and creamy choc coconut mousse. Sometimes I like to combine the coconut meat and avocado as they make a great combination of healthy fats.

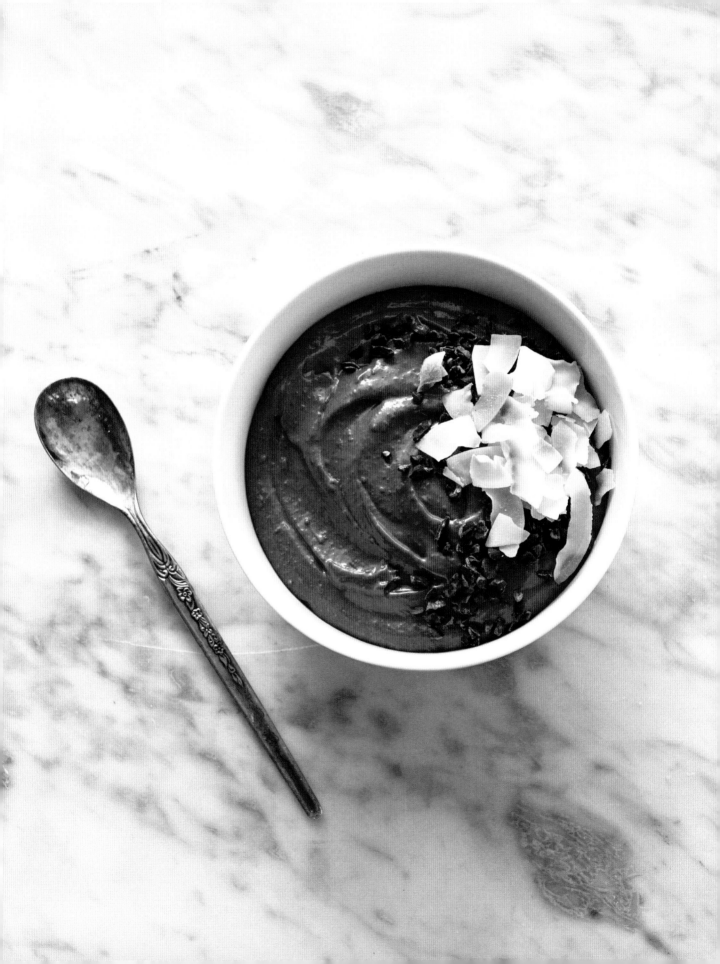

MOCHA MAGIC BITES

BASE

1 cup pecans

3 tbs raw cacao powder

8 Medjool dates

Pinch of pink salt

COFFEE VANILLA CREAM

8 cups raw cashews, soaked

1 tsp vanilla essence

1 1/3 cup Coconut Magic coconut oil, melted

1 cup Coconut Magic coconut nectar

1/2 teaspoon salt

1 1/3 cup very strong, brewed organic coffee

1 cup cacao nibs

CHOCOLATE SAUCE

½ cup cacao powder

½ cup Coconut Magic coconut oil, melted

¼ cup Coconut Magic coconut nectar

½ tsp vanilla essence

Pinch of pink salt

Base:

To make the base, blend the pecans and cacao powder in a food processor, process until a fine flour forms, then add the Medjool dates and salt, and blend again until a sticky dough forms.

Press the mixture into a flat tray or plate lined with a piece of waxed baking paper. Set aside in the fridge.

Coffee Vanilla Cream:

Blend all ingredients.

Pour half of the Coffee Vanilla Cream over the top of the base and refrigerate the remaining half of the cream.

Chocolate Sauce:

Blend all the ingredients for the Chocolate Sauce.

Drizzle the Chocolate Sauce over the top of the Coffee Vanilla Cream, place in freezer and allow to set for 1 hour

Once the chocolate sauce has set, place another layer of the remaining Coffee Vanilla Cream over the top of the chocolate topping layer. Return to the freezer for another 2-3 hours.

Remove from the freezer and slice into bite-size pieces.

Serves approx. 15 square bites + prep: 25 min.. cooling: 4-6 hr.

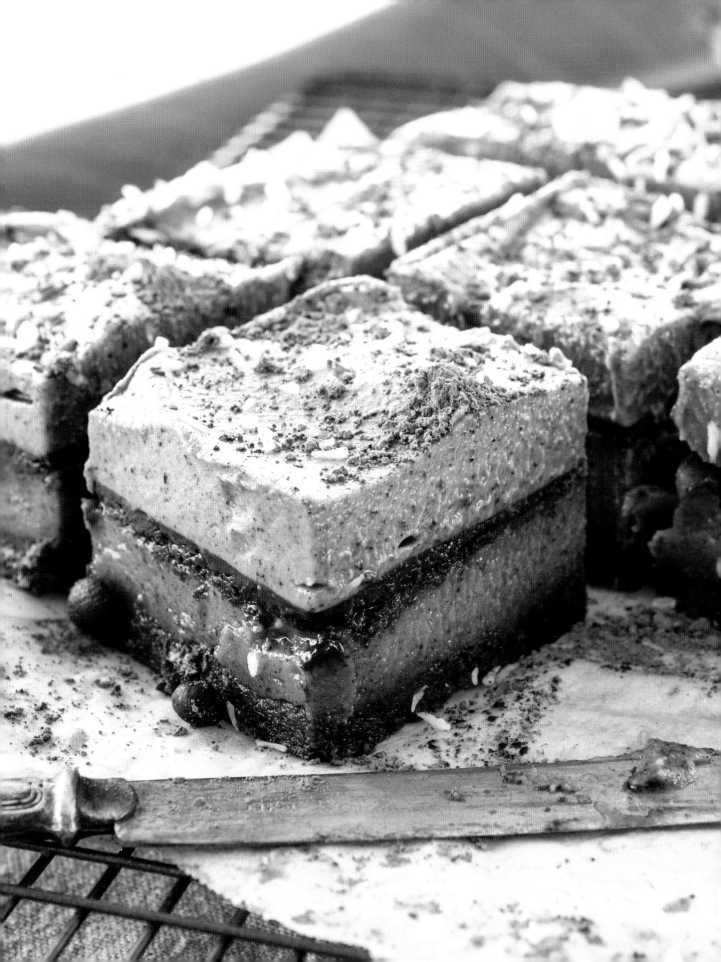

CHERRY CHOC SLICE

BASE

10 x Medjool dates, pitted
and soaked for 4 hours

¼ cup flax seeds

¼ cup sunflower seeds

1 tbs maca powder

2 tbs cacao powder

¼ tsp vanilla bean powder

FILLING

1 cup Coconut Magic
desiccated coconut

¾ cup Coconut Magic coconut oil

1 ½ cups frozen cherries

1 tbs Coconut Magic coconut nectar

CHOCOLATE TOPPING

½ cup cacao powder

½ cup Coconut Magic coconut oil, melted

¼ cup Coconut Magic coconut nectar

Pinch vanilla bean powder

Pinch of pink salt

Base:

Blend all ingredients in a food processor until it forms a ball.

Press the mixture into a pan lined with baking paper and refrigerate,

Filling:

Process all ingredients until well combined. This forms the second layer of the slice – press this on top of the base. Return slice to fridge.

Chocolate Topping:

Blend all ingredients. This makes the third layer of the slice.

Return slice to fridge or freezer for a few minutes before slicing into narrow pieces.

Serves 10 – 12 slices + prep: 30 min.
cooling: 10 – 15 min. soaking: 4 hr.

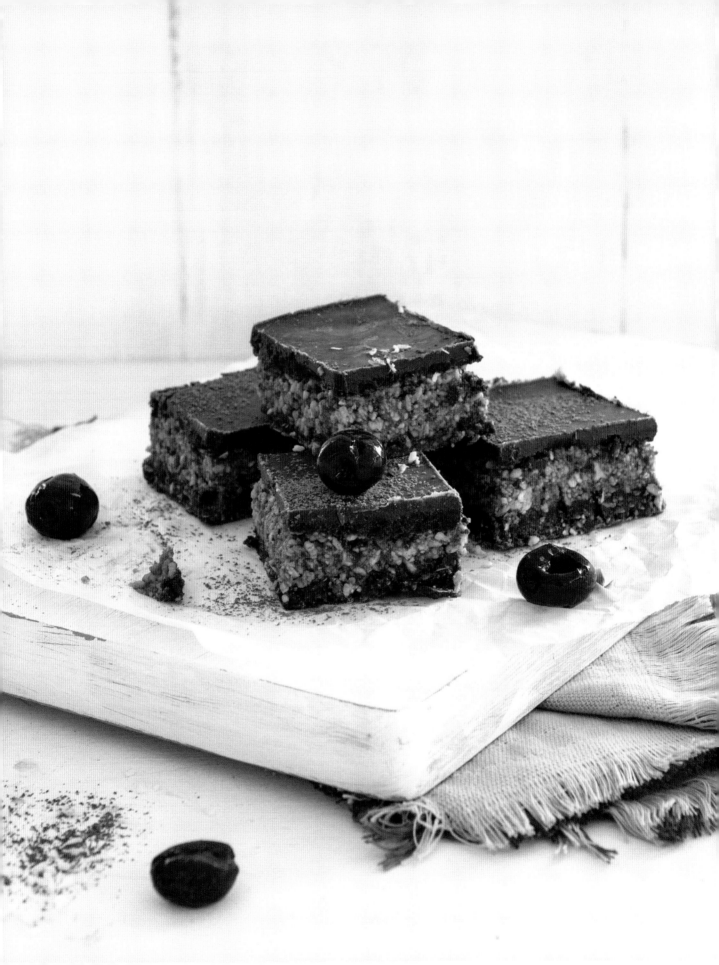

ORANGE CHOCOLATE MOUSSE CAKE

BASE

½ cup raw almonds

½ cup raw walnuts

1 cup pitted Medjool dates

¼ cup Coconut Magic coconut oil, melted

1 tsp vanilla powder

MOUSSE

3 avocados

½ cup Coconut Magic coconut oil

½ cup cacao powder

1 orange, fruit and zest
(or 6 drops food-grade orange essential oil)

½ cup Coconut Magic coconut nectar

¼ tsp cinnamon powder

Pinch of salt

Cacao nibs and orange slices to garnish

Base:

Process the nuts in food processor to a crumbly consistency.

Pulse in coconut oil and vanilla.

Add dates one at a time until well combined and mixture sticks to itself when pressed.

Press into the bottom of a spring-form pan and set aside.

Mousse:

Blend all of the Mousse ingredients in a high-speed blender/food processor until smooth and creamy.

Spread over the base, sprinkle with cacao nibs and refrigerate at least 2-3 hours before serving.

Serves 8-10 slices + prep: 25 min. cooling: 2-3 hr.

Take note...

You can replace avocado with coconut flesh for the filling. Or sometimes I also like to use half coconut flesh and half avocado combined, as they make a great combination of healthy fats!

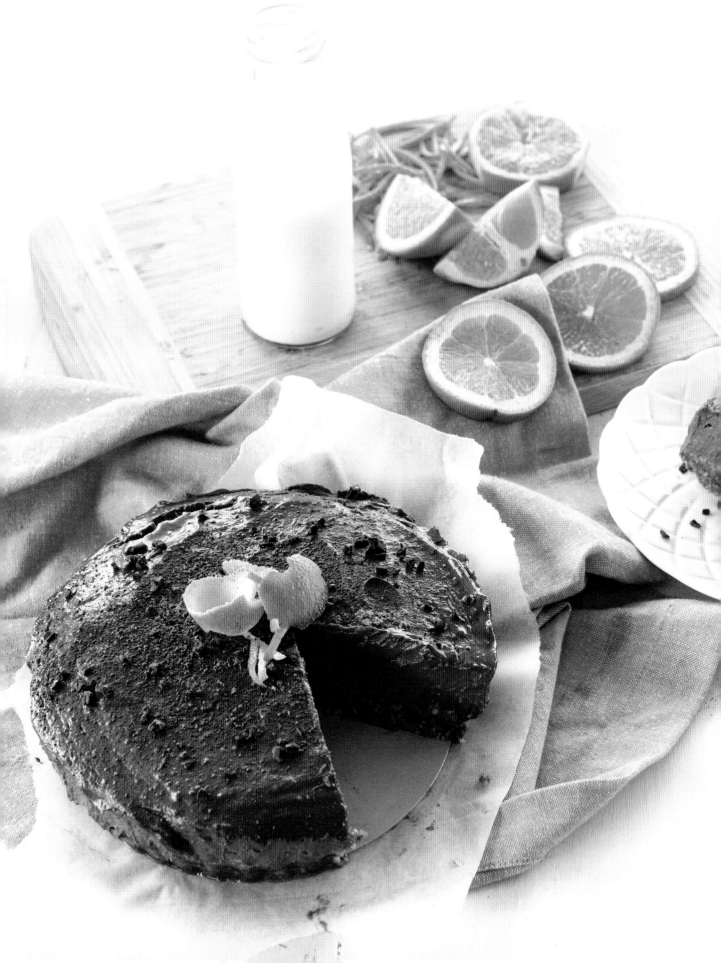

CHOCOLATE FRUIT PIE

BASE

2 whole bananas, sliced

½ whole papaya, sliced
(or mango if you prefer)

CHOCOLATE CREAM

Pinch of vanilla essence

1 cup cashews, soaked at least 2 hours

¼ cup pecan nuts, soaked

½ cup coconut water

1 tbs Coconut Magic coconut oil, melted

1 tbs Coconut Magic coconut nectar

1 tbs cacao powder

Pinch pink salt

Base:

Layer the banana and the papaya/mango into a pie dish or tray. Press gently with your hands, for a few seconds only, to form the base.

Chocolate Cream:

Blend all Chocolate Cream ingredients until smooth and pour over the fruit base.

Decorate with more fruit (optional) and refrigerate for 2 hours before serving.

Serves 2 + prep: 15 min. cooling: 2 hr. soaking: 2 hr.

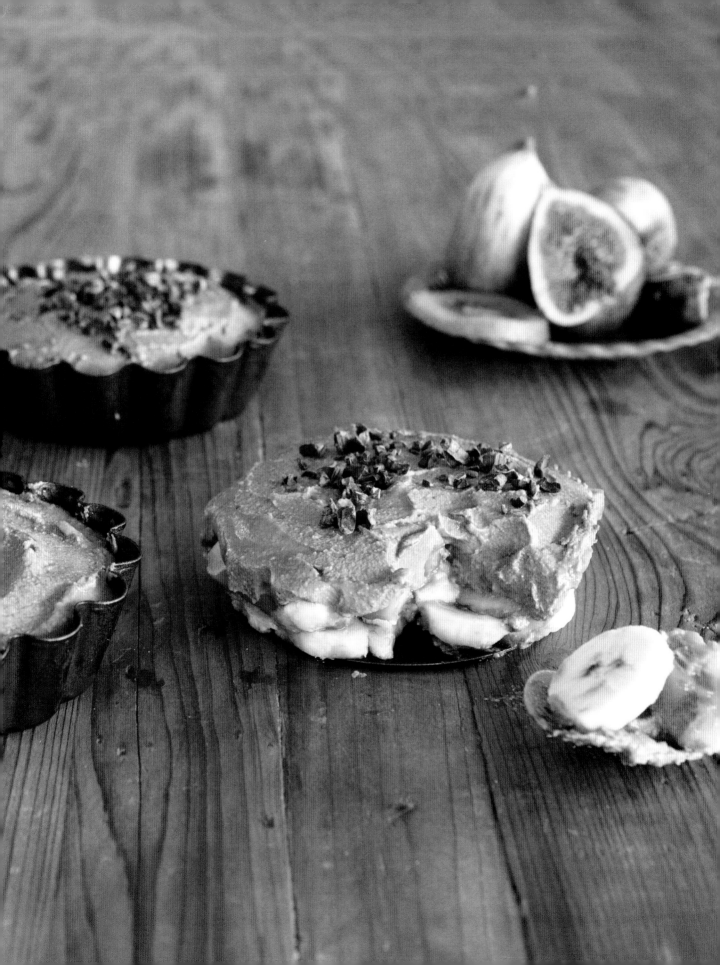

healthy desserts

RAW COCONUT ICE-CREAM WITH RASPBERRY SAUCE

I recommend you buy fresh, young Thai coconuts – not the old brown ones. There is a skill to getting the meat out of the coconuts, and there are many YouTube videos devoted to showing you how!

COCONUT ICE-CREAM

2 cups fresh coconut meat

1 cup coconut water

2 cups raw cashews, soaked for 2hrs then drained

¼ cup Coconut Magic coconut nectar

½ cup Coconut Magic coconut oil, melted

1 tbs vanilla extract

½ tsp pink salt

GARNISH

Coconut Magic coconut flakes

Coconut Magic coconut nectar to garnish (optional)

RASPBERRY SAUCE

1 cup of fresh or frozen raspberries

1 tbs Coconut Magic coconut nectar

Coconut Ice-cream:

Place coconut meat and coconut water in a blender and mix until smooth. Remove from blender and set aside.

Place rinsed and drained cashews in the blender, add just enough of the newly blended coconut mixture to cover the cashews, and blend.

Add remaining ingredients and the rest of the coconut blend. Process until smooth.

Place the mixture into a glass bowl and freeze for a few hours.

You can then add the mixture to an ice-cream maker and churn. If you don't have an ice-cream maker, simply scoop and serve.

Remove the ice-cream from the freezer 10 minutes before serving.

Optional Raspberry Sauce:

This makes your dish look beautiful, it creates some lovely colour and also gives the recipe a sweet raspberry flavour.

Blend raspberries and Coconut Magic coconut nectar together until smooth. Drizzle over the top of your ice-cream.

Serves 6-8 + prep: 20 min. + freeze: 1-2 hrs.

Optional

You can add natural fruit or superfoods for a variety of flavours each time you make this ice-cream. I have made this before with passionfruit, berries and raw cacao powder.

NB: If using frozen raspberries, gently heat the raspberries and nectar in a medium-sized pan over a low heat. Mash the raspberries with a wooden spoon until they become a liquid. Add some lemon juice.

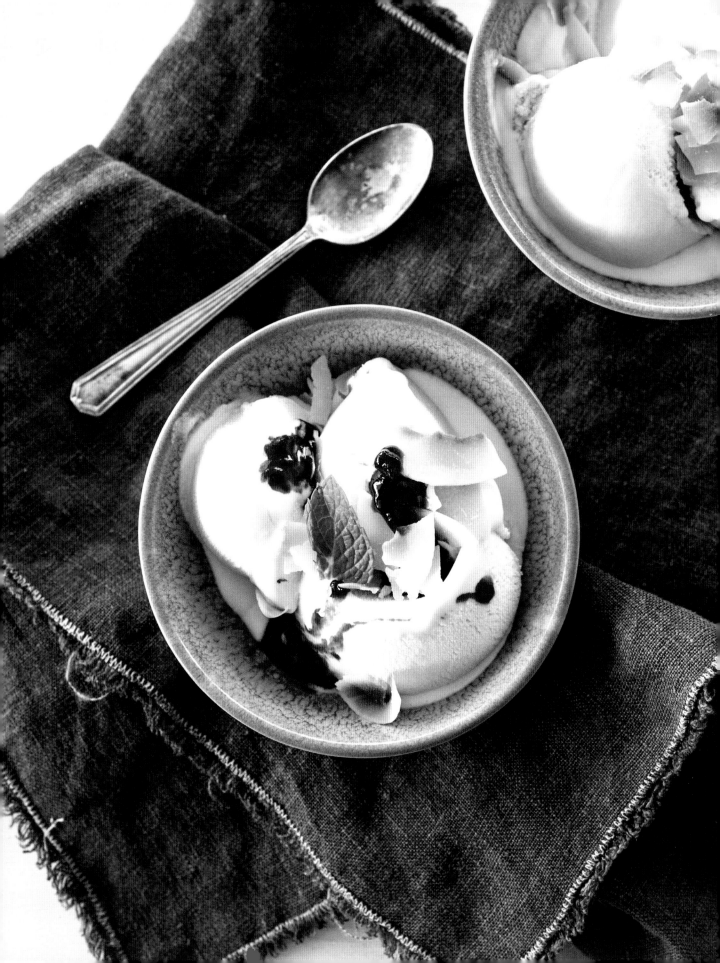

COCONUT & LIME CHEESECAKE

BASE

½ cup of almonds

2 tbs Coconut Magic desiccated coconut

¾ cup of Medjool dates, soaked in warm water for about 15 minutes. Drain well before using.

TOPPING

1 ½ cups of raw cashews, soaked in filtered cold water for a minimum of 4 hours (overnight works best)

½ cup fresh lime juice

Zest of one lime

3 tbs Coconut Magic coconut oil, melted

2 tbs Coconut Magic coconut nectar

½ cup organic coconut milk

The Base:

Add almonds, desiccated coconut and dates to the food processor and pulse into a fine grain.

Lightly grease an 8-inch pan or baking dish with coconut oil.

Press the mixture into the pan until it is well compacted and even. Refrigerate to set.

The Topping:

Rinse and drain the soaked cashews using filtered water.

Combine cashews, lime juice, lime zest, coconut oil, coconut nectar and coconut milk in the blender. Blend well until the mixture is creamy; scrape down the sides as required.

Pour the creamy mixture onto the base, spread evenly and sprinkle with lime zest.

Store in the freezer for an hour or two, or until the cake becomes solid. Remove from freezer 30 minutes before serving.

Serves 6-8 + prep: 30 min. setting: 90 min.

Preparation tips

Soak the cashews in cold water for a minimum of 4 hours. Overnight works best.

Soak the dates in warm water for about 15 minutes. Drain well before using.

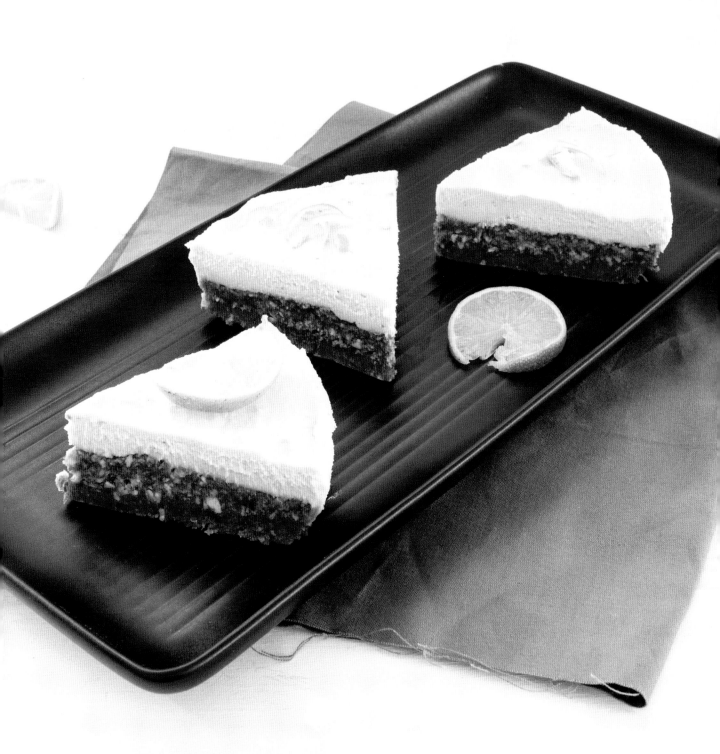

RAW APPLE PIE WITH COCONUT CREAM

CRUST

½ cup pecan nuts, soaked

½ cup walnuts

¼ cup dark raisins

½ cup dried brown figs

2 tbs Coconut Magic coconut oil

Pinch of pink salt

Pinch of nutmeg

FILLING

2 whole apples, peeled and quartered

¼ cup brown figs, chopped

¼ cup pecan nuts, chopped

½ tsp cinnamon powder

½ tsp Coconut Magic coconut nectar

¼ cup Coconut Magic coconut oil

Pinch of pink salt

1 tbs flaxseed powder, ground

1 tbs Coconut Magic coconut flakes

Crust:

Process all crust ingredients in a food processor until almost smooth but still a little chunky.

Then press into an 18 cm round pie tray and refrigerate.

Filling:

Combine all filling ingredients in a blender until smooth.

Pour over the crust.

Decorate with figs, walnuts and coconut flakes.

Refrigerate for at least 2 hours before serving.

Serve with Coconut Cream, see page 113 for the recipe

Serves 6 + prep: 15 min. setting: 2 hrs.

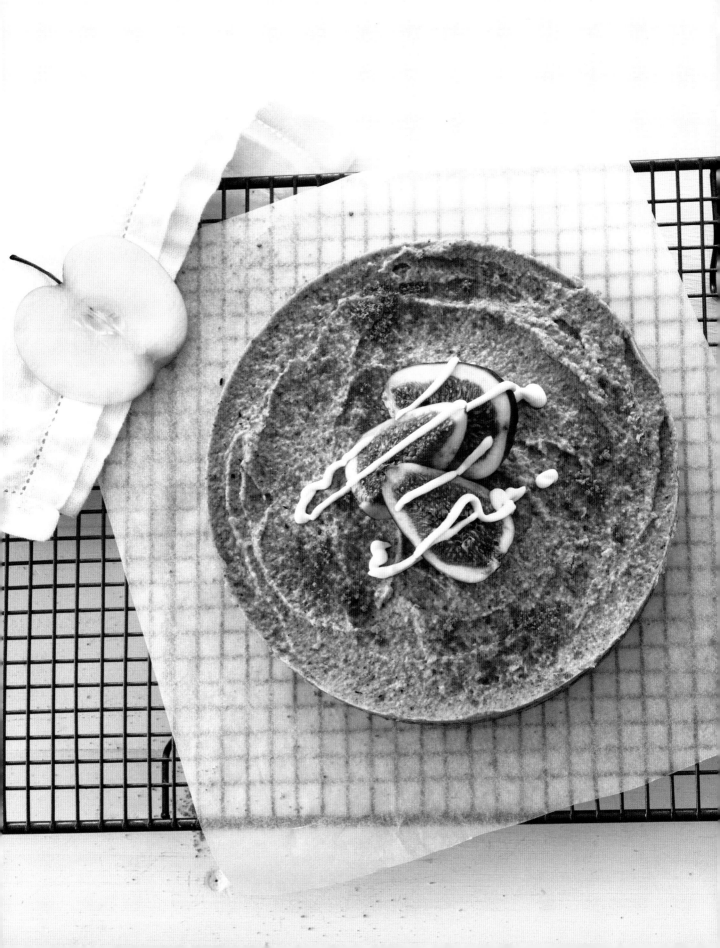

LEMON & COCONUT NUT-FREE SLICE

Caroline Edgar frequently contributes her creative recipes to our blog page. This one was particularly popular because it offered a nut-free raw dessert option.

BASE

1 cup Coconut Magic coconut flakes

½ cup sunflower seeds

10 Medjool dates, chopped in half

1 tbs Coconut Magic coconut nectar

1 tbs tahini

1 tsp lemon zest

TOPPING

2 cups Coconut Magic desiccated coconut or ½ cup coconut butter

½ cup lemon juice

1 large banana, mashed

¼ cup Coconut Magic coconut nectar

1 tbs tahini

¼ cup Coconut Magic coconut oil, melted

½ tsp vanilla powder

1 tbs lucuma powder (optional)

¼ tsp turmeric powder (for an added yellow colour)

Pinch of pink salt

1 tbs poppy seeds (optional)

Base:

Line a 23 x 23 cm tray with baking paper.

In a food processor pulse the coconut flakes until fine (but not as fine as desiccated coconut). Add sunflower seeds and blend again until it all crumbles together. Add the dates and blend until the mixture sticks together.

Add the coconut nectar, tahini and zest to help the mixture stick together.

Press the mixture onto the baking paper – as thick or as thin as you prefer. Set aside in the fridge while you prepare the topping.

Topping:

Blend the desiccated coconut in a food processor for 10-12 minutes until it turns into a liquid. This becomes ½ cup of coconut butter. (If you are using commercial coconut butter, melt in a bowl over warm water until liquid.)

Blend in the lemon juice, banana, coconut nectar and tahini until the mixture is thick yet smooth and creamy.

Add in the melted coconut oil, vanilla powder, lucuma and turmeric with a pinch of salt until it's all combined.

Turn off the blender and stir in the poppy seeds (if using).

Smooth the mixture onto the base, and allow to set for at least 4 hours before slicing. Top with extra coconut flakes and lemon zest.

Store in the fridge for up to a week, or in the freezer and remove half an hour before eating. Enjoy the sweetness with a touch of tang!

Serves 8 + prep: 20 min. setting: 4 hr.

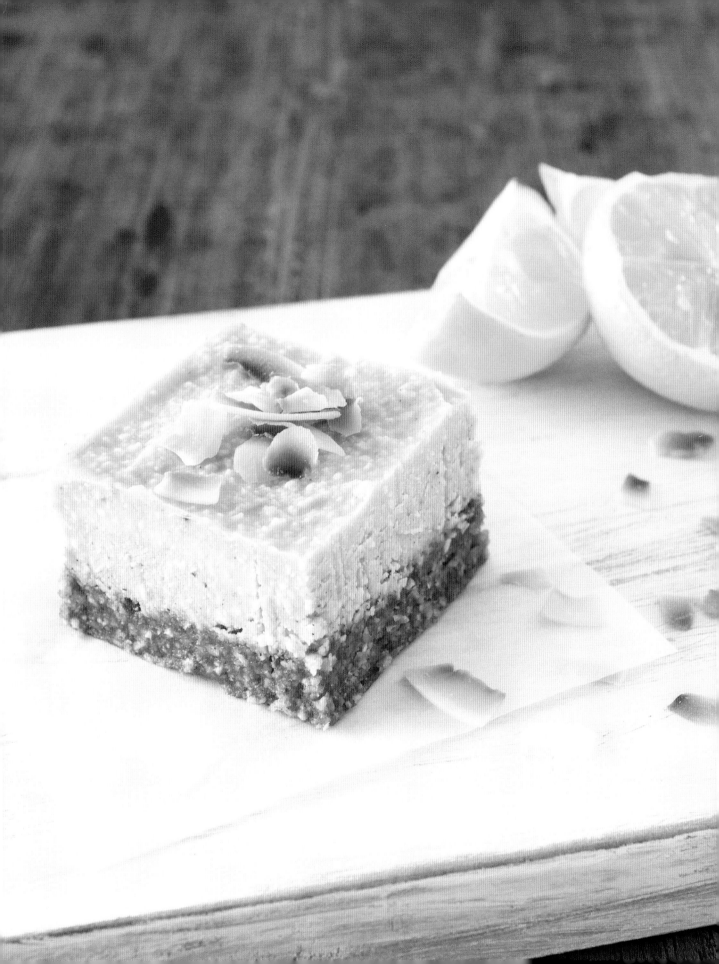

BERRY BLISS BARS

The blueberry is a powerhouse of antioxidants and nutrition, and when combined with coconut provides an awesome pot of goodness for your body.

1 cup coconut butter

1 cup organic blueberries, washed and drained

2 tbs Coconut Magic coconut oil

¼ cup Coconut Magic coconut nectar

2 tsp vanilla essence

Combine all ingredients in a food processor until the mixture is smooth.

Line a 23 x 23 cm pan with parchment paper, leaving some paper sticking out over the sides.

Put the mixture into the pan and spread it out evenly. The mixture is very thick and you may need to use a wet spatula to help spread it evenly.

Gently press down using the extra sides of parchment paper. The paper will lay flat as the mixture is pressed down.

Refrigerate for about 15-20 minutes.

Cut into medium-size pieces and serve!

Store in the fridge in a sealed container for up to two weeks.

Makes 12 medium size pieces + prep: 20 min. setting: 20 min.

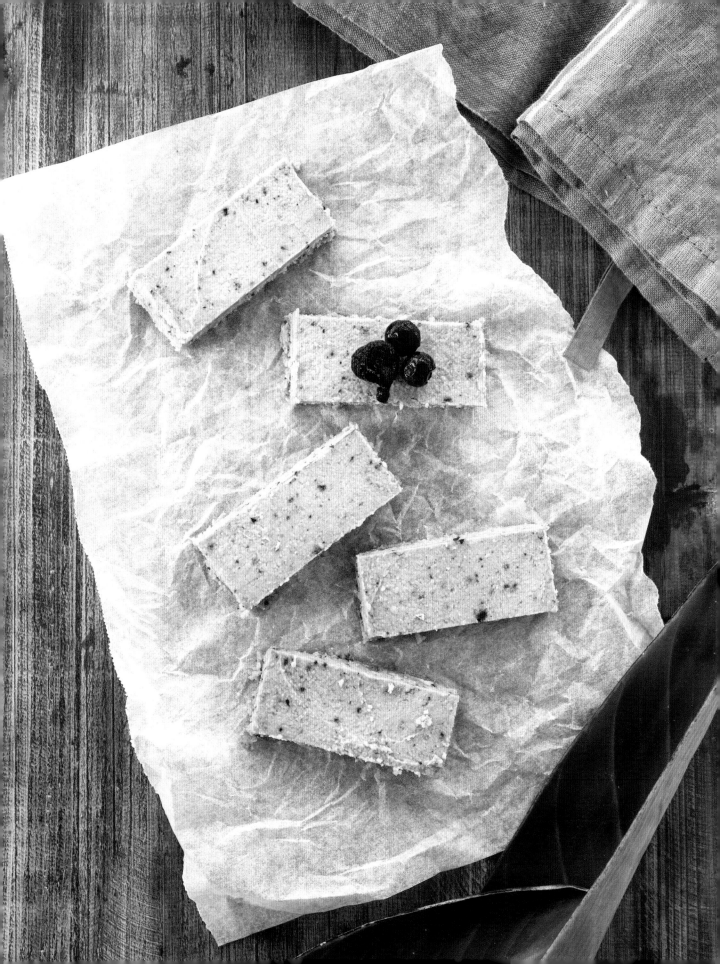

ACAI BERRY COCONUT ICE-CREAM

4 cups coconut milk

¼ cup Coconut Magic coconut sugar

2 cups frozen acai pulp (unsweetened)

1 large banana

1 cup organic frozen blueberries, washed and drained

2 tbs Coconut Magic coconut oil

Combine all ingredients in a blender and process until smooth.

Transfer contents of blender to an airtight container and store in your freezer, until solid. Overnight usually works best.

Remove from the freezer and allow to thaw for 5-10 minutes before serving.

Top with some fresh berries, crushed nuts and coconut flakes.

For added sweetness you can also drizzle some coconut nectar on top of your ice-cream.

Keeps in the freezer for up to 3 weeks.

Serves 10 + prep: 15 min.
freeze: 3-4 hours, overnight is best.

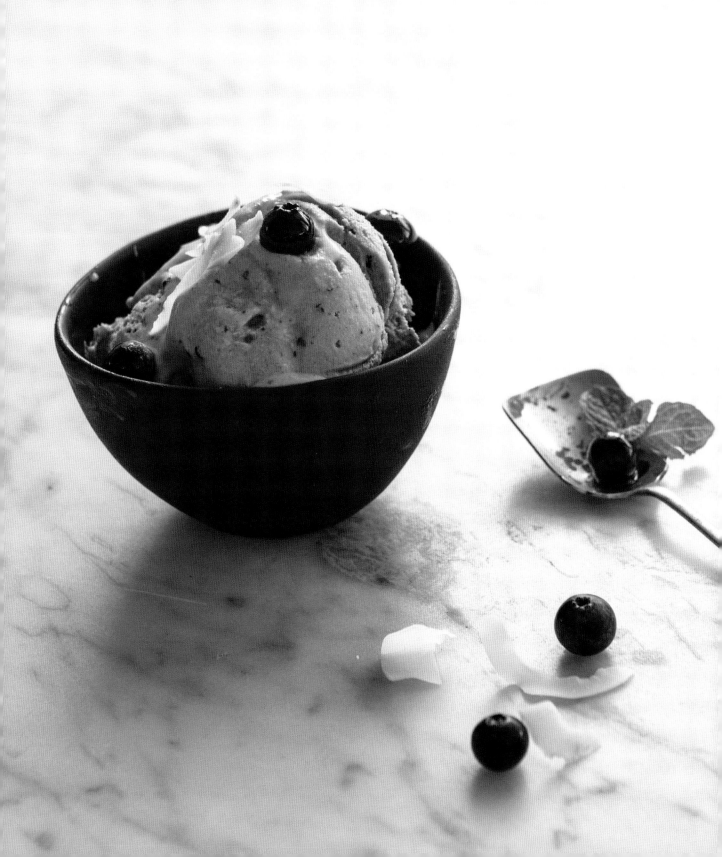

CHOC ALMOND BLISS BALLS

½ cup cacao butter

¼ cup cacao powder

1½ cups almond meal

¼ cup Coconut Magic coconut nectar

8 Medjool dates, seeds removed

½ tsp vanilla essence

Pinch of pink salt

¼ tsp cinnamon

Melt the cacao butter.

Place all ingredients into food processor and mix well until a smooth paste is formed.

Roll into balls.

Refrigerate for one hour and serve.

Makes 8 – 10 balls + prep: 20 min. setting: 1 hr.

COCONUT ROUGH BLISS BALLS

2 cups Coconut Magic desiccated coconut

2 cups of walnuts

Pinch pink salt

8 Medjool dates, seeds removed

¼ cup cacao powder

2 tbs Coconut Magic coconut oil, melted

2 tbs cacao butter, melted

Pinch vanilla essence

2 tsp Coconut Magic coconut sugar

Blend 1 ½ cups of Coconut Magic desiccated coconut, walnuts and salt in the food processor until finely ground.

Add the dates and process until the mixture becomes sticky.

Add all other ingredients (except the remainder of the desiccated coconut) and process until well combined. Roll into balls of bliss!

Coat the balls with the remainder of the desiccated coconut. Refrigerate for one hour and serve.

Makes 8 – 10 balls + prep: 20 min. setting: 1 hr.

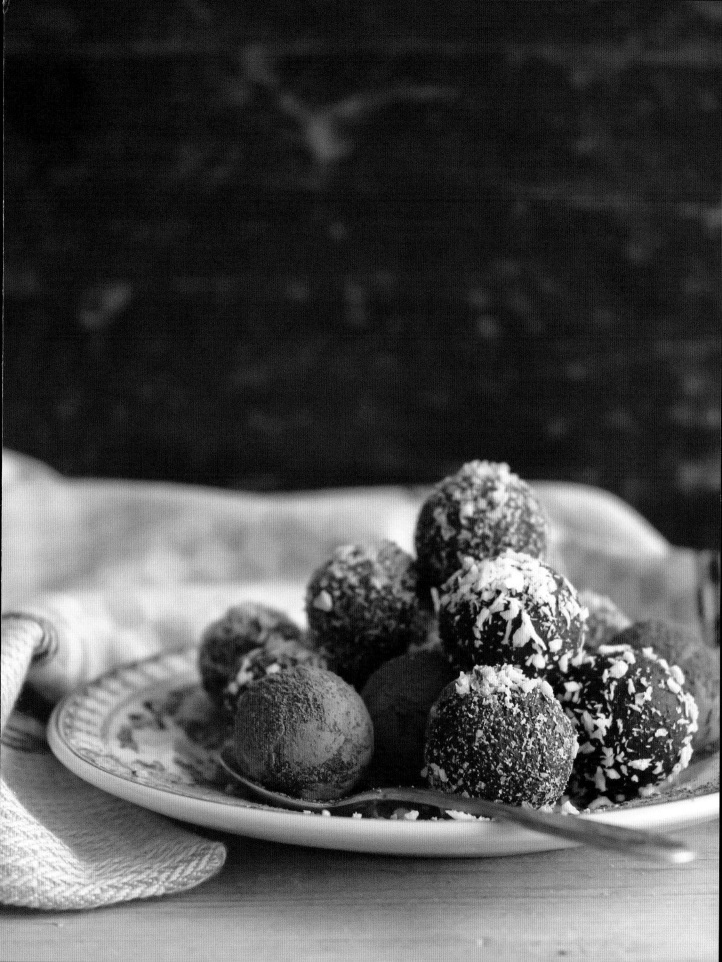

AVOCADO & COCONUT POPSICLES

2 ripe avocados

1 ½ cups organic coconut milk

¼ cup Coconut Magic coconut oil

¼ cup Coconut Magic coconut nectar

2 tsp freshly squeezed lime juice

1 tsp vanilla extract

Combine all ingredients in a blender or food processor and blend until creamy.

Pour into popsicle molds.

Freeze for 1½ to 2 hours. Enjoy!

serves 4-6 + prep: 5 min. + freeze: 2 hrs.

Tip

Run popsicles under warm water to remove smoothly!

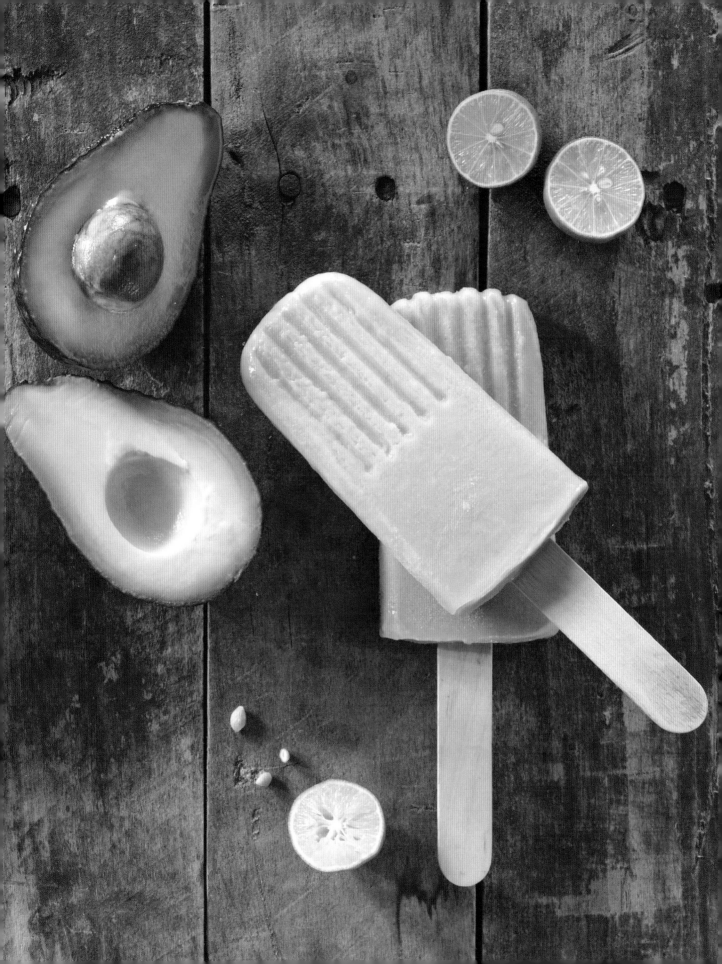

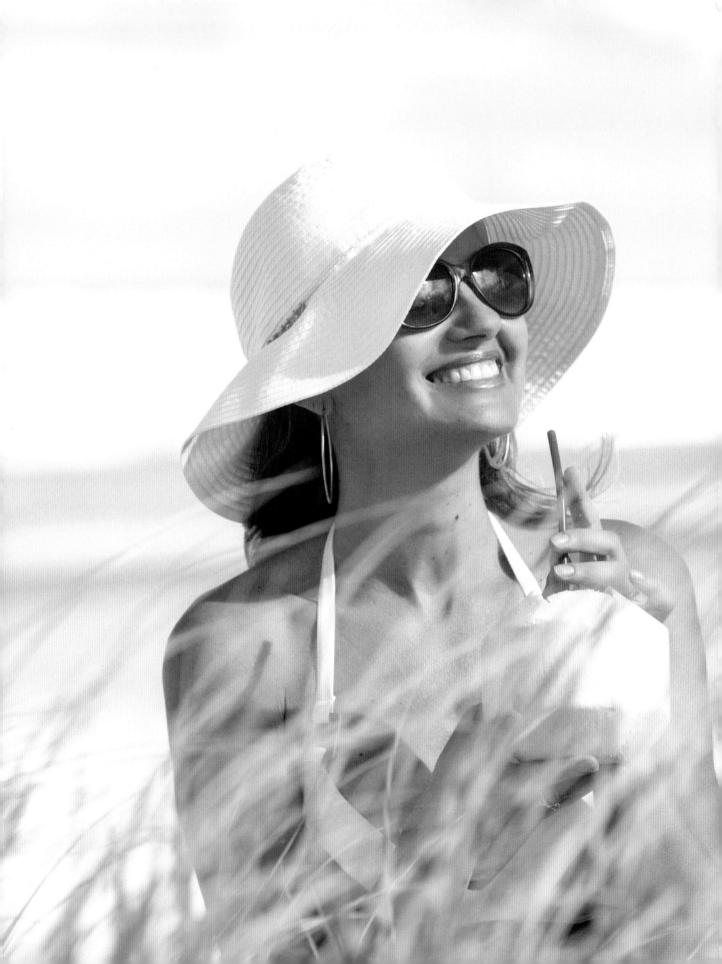

coconut
body care
& beauty

Coconut oil has been used for thousands of years in many cultures to promote beauty and good health, thanks to its high concentration of medium chain fatty acids.

Taken internally and applied externally, coconut oil gives you the best of both worlds, so you can look and feel good on the inside, and on the outside.

Used topically, coconut oil gives you a very natural, organic and toxic-free body and health care regime.

Here are some great recipes for body care and beauty:

CINNAMON LIP BALM

1 tbs cacao butter

1 tbs candelilla wax (optional)

1½ tbs Coconut Magic coconut oil

3 drops cinnamon essential oil

Grate the cacao butter and candelilla wax into a stainless steel bowl.

Using a double boiler melt the wax and the butter, stirring to help blend together. Add the coconut oil and stir until all ingredients are melted and well blended.

Remove the bowl from the boiler and add the drops of essential oil. Pour into a glass jar or a small tin. Label the jar so you know what's in it!

COCONUT OIL DEODORANT

¼ cup of baking soda, aluminium free

¼ cup arrowroot powder

¼ cup Coconut Magic coconut oil, melted

10 drops of essential oil (lavender, lemon, frankincense, tea tree and rosemary all work well. Or you can create your own blend).

Mix the powdered ingredients in a bowl.

Add the coconut oil, mixing well.

Add the essential oils

Store in a small container or a mason jar. Use your fingers to apply the deodorant under your arms.

COCO BODY SCRUB

½ cup Coconut Magic coconut oil

1 cup Coconut Magic coconut sugar

8-10 drops lavender essential oil (optional)

Using a whisk, beat the coconut oil for a few minutes, add the coconut sugar and essential oil (if using) and whisk a little more until everything is blended together.

CACAO BODY BUTTER

½ cup cacao butter, melted

¼ cup Coconut Magic coconut oil, melted

⅛ cup sweet almond oil

½ tsp vitamin E oil

Melt the cacao butter in a double boiler (or melt in a small saucepan which is placed inside a larger saucepan filled with boiling water.)

Add the coconut oil.

Add all other ingredients and mix well.

Store in a container with a sealed lid. Use as required after a shower or bath.

NB: you can also add some essential oils for added aroma. Orange and cinnamon go well with the lovely chocolate fragrance from the cacao butter.

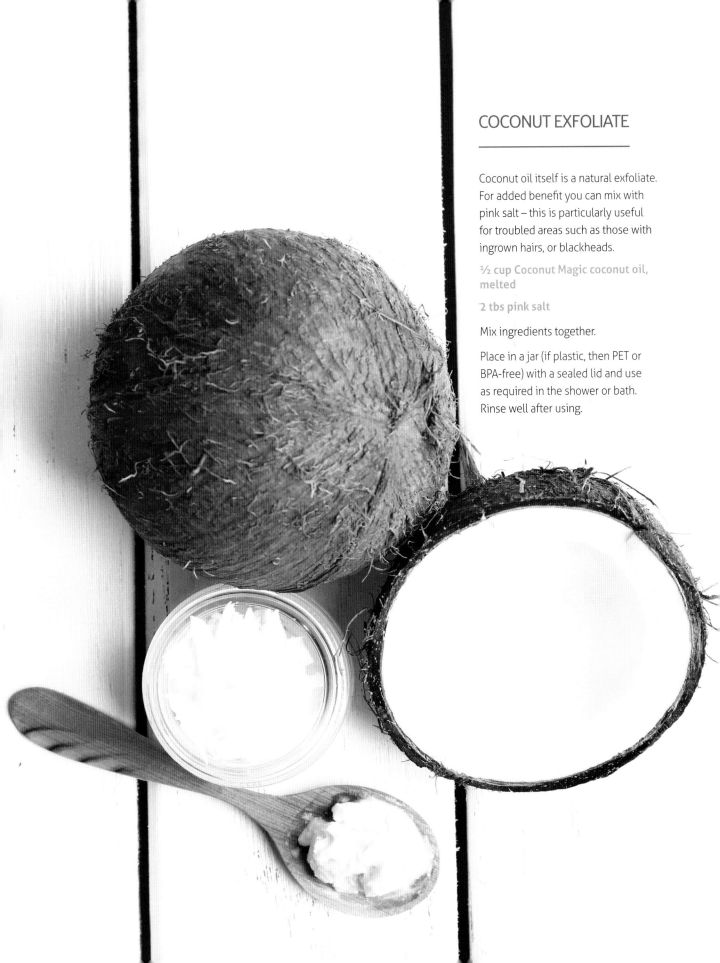

COCONUT EXFOLIATE

Coconut oil itself is a natural exfoliate. For added benefit you can mix with pink salt – this is particularly useful for troubled areas such as those with ingrown hairs, or blackheads.

½ cup Coconut Magic coconut oil, melted

2 tbs pink salt

Mix ingredients together.

Place in a jar (if plastic, then PET or BPA-free) with a sealed lid and use as required in the shower or bath. Rinse well after using.

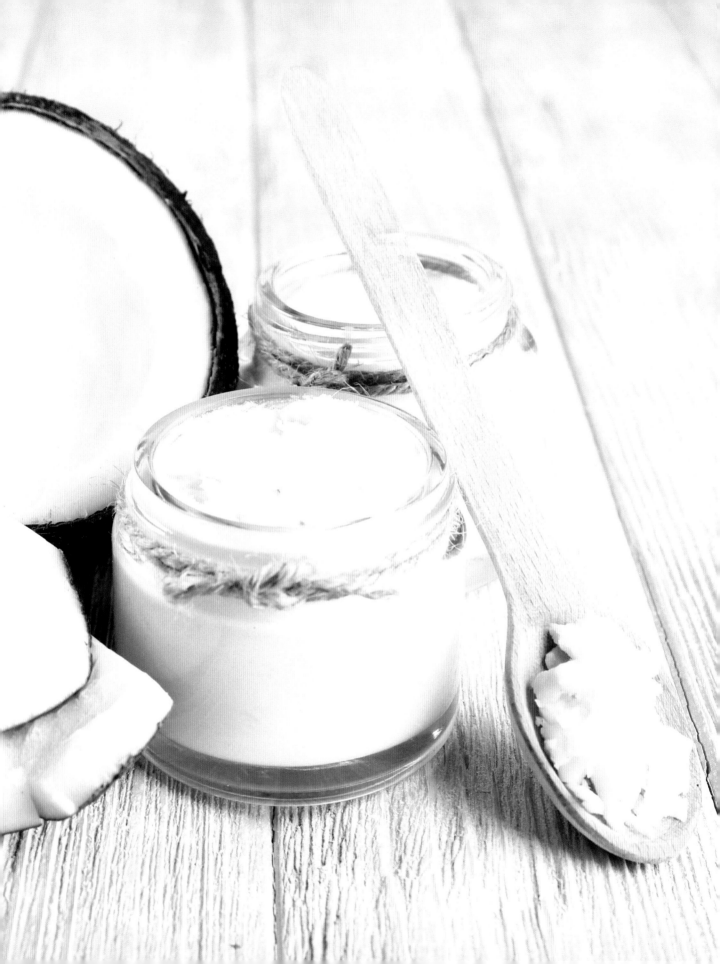

COCONUT OIL TOOTHPASTE

The natural anti-bacterial and anti-fungal properties in coconut oil benefit oral health and hygiene, and help keep teeth clean and white.

I have come across a few ingredients in toothpaste that claim to help with oral and dental health, when in fact they can cause further issues.

1. Glycerin: this gives toothpaste its creamy texture. It is also meant to assist teeth with 'protection', but at the same time it stops re-enamalisation (so cavities are unable to self heal).

2. Sodium fluoride: this is a by-product of aluminium manufacturing. It can also be found in rat poison and industrial pesticides.

An easy solution to a healthy and safe toothpaste is to make your own with coconut oil. You can even adjust the recipe to suit your own taste, make it sweet, minty or fruity.

3 tbs Coconut Magic coconut oil, melted

3 tbs baking soda

8 drops essential oil (peppermint, cinnamon and orange are good)

1 tsp stevia or xylitol (optional for sweetening)

Mix the powdered ingredients in a bowl.

Add the melted coconut oil – roughly divide the oil into three parts and add one part at a time. Mix well. Add the essential oils.

Store in a small container or a mason jar and use a spoon or popsicle stick to spoon out the toothpaste as required.

TREATING CELLULITE

Cellulite is one of the hardest types of fats to dissolve in the body. Cellulite is an accumulation of old fat cell clusters that solidify and harden as the surrounding tissue loses its elasticity.

Tangerine, orange and lemon essential oils actually help reduce fat cells. Grapefruit essential oil is fat-dissolving and also detoxifies.

Simply add 1-2 drops of your favourite citrus blend of essential oil to a small amount of coconut oil and massage into the affected areas. I like to use a 25 ml or 150 ml jar of Coconut Magic coconut oil, add my essential oils to the jar, and use it daily.

Another great benefit of using coconut oil and essential oils is that it may also help to prevent stretch marks!

Take note...

Please note that although citrus oils are great to break down cellulite and tone the skin, they also enhance the photosynthesising effect of the sun. Avoid applying citrus oils to skin that will be exposed to direct sunlight or UV light within 24 hours or make sure to keep those parts covered.

You should begin to see results in 4-6 weeks. You can also support this detox by including citrus fruits such as grapefruit and lemon in your diet. Juicing is a good way to do this. A three-day grapefruit juice fast is known to have tremendous results for treating cellulite.

COCONUT BATH TIME

Add a generous amount of coconut oil to the bath and literally soak in its moisturising effects. This can be combined with some Epsom salts to soothe muscles, and your favourite essential oil blends.

Coconut oil is safe to use in baths for babies and children. It will benefit their skin too.

A woman once shared on our Facebook page that she took a 'coconut oil' bath three times per week during her pregnancy to avoid stretch marks, and it worked!

HAIR CONDITIONING TREATMENT

Since ancient times coconut oil has been used as the preferred hair treatment in areas such as India, Sri Lanka, Thailand, Burma, Malaysia and the Caribbean, with remarkable results. Certain components in it keep the hair strong, nourished and protected from the effects of premature ageing, like baldness and excessive hair loss.

Coconut oil has a high moisture retaining capacity; it is not easily broken down nor does it evaporate, which makes it very stable. This keeps hair moist and soft, which prevents hair breakage.

Apply warm or melted coconut oil straight to your hair. Massage your scalp and ensure all ends are covered. Leave the oil in your hair as a treatment for at least 4 hours. I find that overnight works best.

Place a towel over your pillow so the oil doesn't get onto your pillow case.

Optional: Brunettes and redheads use 5 drops of rosemary essential oil, and chamomile for blondes.

COCONUT OIL FACE WASH

1 tbs Coconut Magic coconut oil

Optional: 2-3 drops of essential oil (lavender and frankincense work well)

Optional: For oily skin also use a squeeze of lemon juice.

Mix all ingredients together well. If you do this in your hand the coconut oil will melt.

Apply to your face and massage into your skin as you would your regular face cleanser.

Leave on for a minute or two and then wipe your face with a damp face cloth.

Rinse with a splash of water and then pat dry with a clean towel.

BODY MOISTURISER

Pure coconut oil can be used on its own or with your favourite essential oils as a full body moisturiser. A small amount goes a long way, so use sparingly. Unlike lotions you don't need to rub coconut oil into your skin, simply apply to your skin and then spread gently with your fingers and hands, allow your skin to naturally soak up the oil. It takes less than a minute to fully absorb.

Depending on your skin requirements, you might like to do this two to three times per week, or even every day.

Coconut oil can also be used in the shower as a moisturising body wash. In the shower apply liberally and massage in. After your shower, gently pat your skin dry with a towel.

Your skin will look and feel amazing!

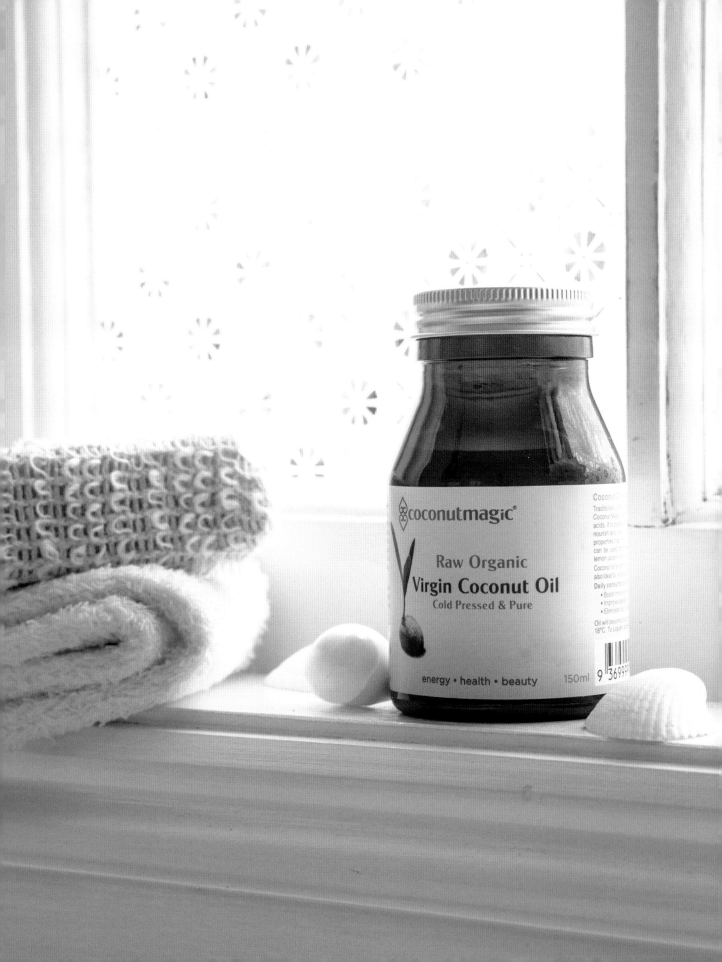

GLOSSARY OF COCONUT MAGIC PRODUCTS

Coconut Aminos

Made from small batches of freshly harvested coconut-flower nectar, coconut amino sauce is a deliciously healthy, wheat- and soy-free alternative to tamari or soy sauce, with 17 important naturally occurring amino acids. Great for salads, dressings, marinades, soups, vegetables, rice and beans, stir-fries, meat, fish and sushi. This product is coming soon and is currently in research and development at Coconut Magic.

Coconut Butter

Coconut butter is creamy with a beautiful coconut flavour. It contains the coconut oil, as well as the fibre and the protein from the coconut meat. Made by drying the coconut flesh with hot air, the dehydrated flesh is then ground into a paste and placed into a vacuum sealed glass jar. This product is coming soon and is currently in research and development at Coconut Magic.

Desiccated Coconut

Organic desiccated coconut is made by simply drying and shredding fresh coconut meat to produce a crisp, snow-white grainy substance that has a sweet, pleasant aroma while retaining the fresh taste of the coconut. It's important to buy dried coconut without added sweeteners or other additives.

Coconut Flakes

Organic coconut flakes have a clean and delicious coconut flavour, with all the benefits of fresh coconut meat. Dried coconut is a rich source of lauric acid (which has anti-microbial properties) in addition to being a great source of dietary fibre and protein. Also known as coconut chips.

Coconut Flour

Coconut flour is made from fresh coconut meat. The meat is dried then finely ground into a powder, very similar in consistency to wheat flour. Coconut Magic organic coconut flour is great as a low-carb, high-fibre, gluten-free alternative to wheat flour, for baking.

Coconut Flower Nectar

Coconut flower nectar is naturally sweet and highly nutritious. Coconut Magic coconut nectar is derived from the liquid sap of coconut flowers. This organic coconut product has a very low glycemic index (35) and contains vitamins, minerals, amino acids and a range of other nutrients.

Coconut Oil

Made cold-pressed, virgin and raw, coconut oil is the elixir of the coconut, the essence of magic extracted from the fresh coconut meat. Coconut oil is one of the few foods that can be classified as a superfood. Its unique combination of fatty acids can have profound positive effects on health. These include fat loss, better brain function and various other amazing benefits. Use for cooking, in smoothies and warm drinks, oil-pulling therapy, skincare and more.

Coconut Sugar

Coconut Magic coconut sugar, produced from coconut palm blossoms, is a delicious and healthy alternative to cane sugar. It has a toffee-like flavour, is natural and organic, has been minimally processed, and has not been filtered. Coconut sugar is crystallised coconut nectar and therefore boasts the same nutritional profile and low glycemic index.

Coconut Vinegar

Coconut vinegar is made from the liquid sap of the coconut tree, the same sap that is used to produce coconut nectar. Coconut Magic coconut vinegar is made from coconut nectar, and is naturally aged for eight months to one year, with no other addition or alteration, thereby fully retaining and even enhancing its nutrient-rich properties as it forms its own 'mother'. Use as an ingredient for salad dressings, recipes and for inner cleansing.

Other Coconut Magic Products :

Raw Energy Bars

Coconut Magic's raw bars were created out of our own desire to eat healthy and raw whilst on the go. Each bar is vegan, gluten-free, Paleo friendly, sugar-free, dairy-free and soy-free, made from 100% whole food and raw food ingredients. Each bar also contains Coconut Magic organic virgin coconut oil and coconut flower nectar, for added health benefits and a delicious taste. Made in Australia from natural ingredients and nothing else.

Varieties include:
Coconut: Dates, Almonds, Coconut, Cashews, Pecans, Coconut Chips, Coconut Nectar, Coconut Oil
Cacao: Dates, Almonds, Cashews, Coconut, Tahini, Cacao, Coconut Oil, Coconut Nectar
Raspberry: Dates, Almonds, Coconut, Goji Berries, Cashews, Raspberry Powder, Coconut Nectar, Coconut Oil
Chai Spice: Dates, Chia Seeds, Sunflower Seeds, Sesame Seeds, Vanilla Bean Extract, Ginger Powder, All Spice, Cinnamon, Cardamom Powder, Coconut Oil

Visit our website for product updates as we are frequently adding to our coconut range: www.coconutmagic.com

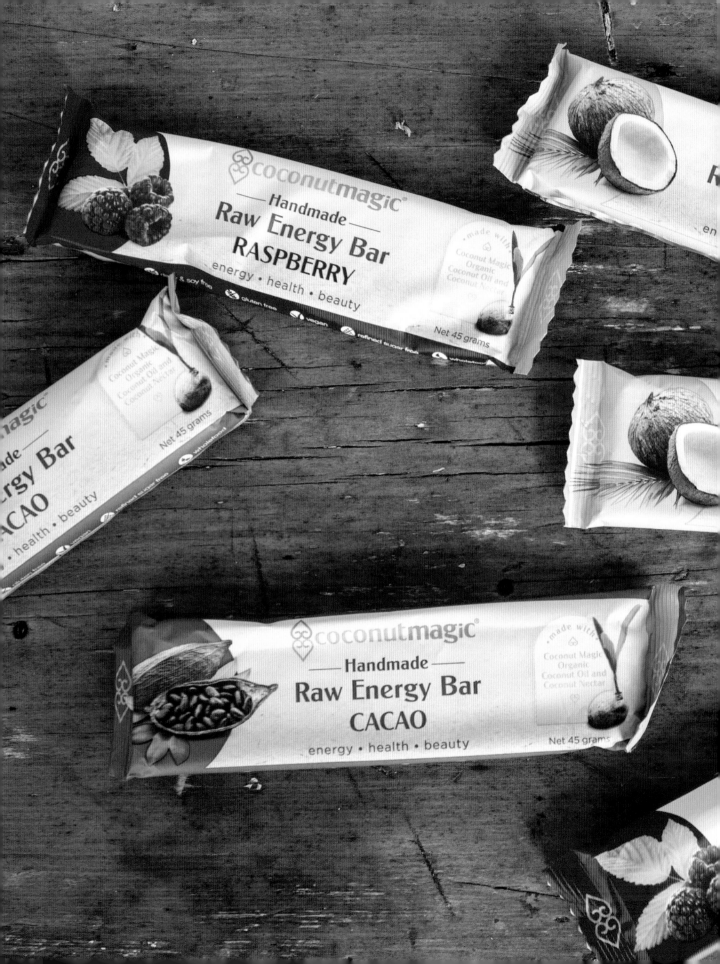

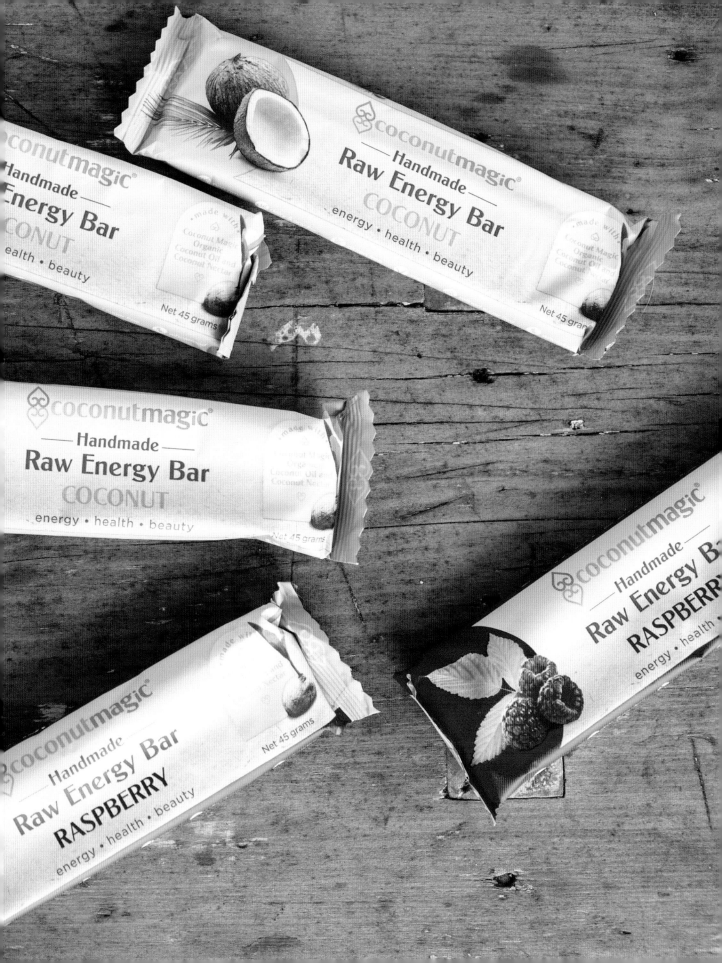

INDEX

A

Acne, 58, 61-64
Almond milk, 40, 44
Alzheimer's, 16, 18, 34, 49-50, 55
Aminos, 24, 44
Amino acids, 25, 61
Antioxidants, 26, 37, 42
Apple pie
    Raw Apple Pie With Coconut Cream, recipe, **208**
Arthritis, 16, 18, 58, (in dogs, 69)
Asparagus; Blanched Asparagus With Flax-Oil Dressing, recipe, 162
Aspartame, 27
Avocado
    Avocado & Coconut Popsicles, recipe, 218
    Avocado & Cucumber Soup, raw, recipe, 128
    Avocado Aioli Dressing, recipe, 182
    Avocado Salsa, recipe, 164

B

Baby massage oil, 54
Basil Sauce, recipe, 144
Bath oils , 34, 53, 54
Berry & Pear Crumble, recipe, 100
Blood sugar, 10, 24, 35, 46, 48
Body scrub, 35
Boost metabolism, 16, 19, 35, 46-47, (when pregnant, 53) 54-55
Brain health, 16, 35, 49-50, (in babies, 53) 55-61.
Brain health recipes: 82, 218, 224, 208
Breakfast Bars, recipe 92
Breast-feeding, 20-21, 35, 53-54
Bruises, 61, 62
Buckwheat Wraps, recipe, 102
Burns, 34
Butter, 17-19, 45
Butters
    Almond Butter, recipe, 110
    Chocolate Butter, recipe, 110
    Coconut Butter, recipe, 110

C

Cacao powder , 39
Calcium, sources of, 26, 40
Cancer, 16, 21, 49, 53, 66, 69
Candida, 12, 20, 35, 44, 49, 54, 56, 57, 66
Candida cleanse, 44, 56
Cane sugar, 24-25, 27
Capric acid, 20, 31, 48
Caprylic acid, 20, 31, 48, 67
Caproic acid, 20
Carrot, Ginger And Sweet Potato Soup, recipe, 118
Cauliflower Rice, recipe, 134
Cauliflower, Roasted, With Coconut + Spice, recipe, 162
Cellulite, 64
Cheesecake; Coconut & Lime Cheesecake, recipe, 206
Cheesy Broccoli snack, recipe, 162
Choc Chia & Hemp Bowl, recipe, 98
Chia Jam, recipe, 104
Chips, Salt & Vinegar Kale Chips, recipe, 160
Cholesterol, 16-18, 20, 25, 39, 55
Cocoa powder, 39
Coconut recipes
    Cinnamon & Coconut Quinoa Porridge, recipe, 96
    Coconut Bread With Chia Jam, recipe, 104
    Coconut Cereal, recipe, page 94
    Coconut Flour Pancakes recipe, 90
    Coconut Ice-Cream, recipe, 204
    Coconut Lentil Curry With Cauliflower Rice, recipe 134
    Coconut Quinoa With Kale & Pesto, recipe, 138
    Coconut Soup, raw, recipe, 126
Coconut meat, 28, 32, 37, 40, 48, 56, 69
Cravings, 9, 34, 35, 47, 49
Coconut oil – for babies, 50, 53, 55, 62
    Baby massage oil, 54
    Cradle cap, 54

Infant health, 20, 21, 49, 53
Nappy rash cream, 54
Premature babies, 53
Teething, 54
Yeast infections/candida, 54
Coconut oil – for beauty
Bath oils, 35
Body scrub, 35
Deodorant, 35, 60, 64, recipe page 226
Exfoliant, 64
Face, 45, 61, 64
Hair, 35, 45, 64, 65, recipe page 229
Lip balm, 35, 45, 64
Moisturiser, 35, 61-62, 64
Stretch marks, 34, 53, 64
Sunscreen, 65
Coconut oil capsules, 36
Coconut oil – for hair, 35, 42, 45, 54, 64-65
Coconut oil – for health
Antioxidants, 28, 46
Blood-sugar balance, 34-35, 46, 48
Body synergy, 64
Brain health, 16, 35, 49-50, (in children, 53), 55
Candida, 20, 35, 44, 49, (in children, 54), 56, 57, 61, 80, 112
Cravings, 9, 34, 35, 47, 49
Cellulite, 64
Crohn's disease, 49, 61
Detoxification, 34, 46-47, 49, 56-57, 58, 64, 66, recipes: 81, 84, 124,
Diabetes. 16, 20, 34, 49, 61, 69,
Environmental toxins, 60
Gallbladder, 19, 40, 46, 49, 61
Healthy digestion and nutrient absorption, 48
Hormones, 18, 35, 47, 54-55, 58,
Liver, 18, 19, 24-25, 46-47, 49, 50, 55
Obesity, 16, 18, 47, 49
Pancreatitis, 49
Thyroid health, 40, (in pregnancy, 53), 54-55
Weight loss, 19, 34, 47, 49, 64
Coconut oil – how much to eat, 34
Coconut oil – for pets, 69
Coconut oil – for pregnancy
Lactation, 53
Stretch marks, 53, 64

Coconut oil – production
Centrifuge – wet milling/vacuum evaporation, 32
Coconut Magic production, 28, 29
Direct Micro Expelling, 32
Expeller pressed, 27
Extraction process , 27, 28, 29, 32, 33
Extra-virgin, 27
Fermentation, 28, 32
Hydrogenated, 27
MCT, 20
Packaging and transportation, 33
Refined, bleached and deodorised, 31
Quick dry, 28
Therapeutic grade, 27-28
Virgin (VCO), 27-31
Coconut oil – for sex
Vaginal health, 67
Lubricant, 67
Coconut oil – for skin
Acne, 58, 61-64
Body scrub, 35
Bruises, 61, 62
Burns, 34
Cellulite, 64
Eczema, 12-13, 61-62
Skin tissue damage, 60
Skin wounds, 61
Coconut oil
Taste and smell, 13, 27-28, 31-33, 36
Weight loss, 19, 34, 47, 49, 64
Coconut sugar, 25-26, 45
Coconut vinegar, 41-42, 57, 66
Coconut water, 33, 45, 48, 56
Coconut yoghurt, 41, 66, 112
Coeliac disease, 41
Cold-sore treatment, 35
Coleslaw + Coconut Citrus Vinaigrette, recipe, 178
Contaminated foods, 42-43
Copra, 31
Corn syrup, 24, 27
Crackers; Coconut & Chia Herbed Crackers, recipe, 158
Cravings, 9, 34, 35, 47, 49
Crohn's disease, 49, 61
Curry; Coconut Lentil Curry With Cauliflower Rice, recipe 134

D

Dairy – the facts, 39
David Gillespie, 16, 24, 70
Deodorant, 35, 60, 64, recipe page 226
Delia McCabe, 70
Dental – see oral hygiene
Detoxification, 34, 46-47, 49, 56-57, 58, 64, 66, recipes: 81, 84, 124, 128
Diabetes, 16, 18, 20, 25, 34, 49, 61, 69,
Diets –
    Paleo, 37
    Raw food, 37
    Superfoods, 37
    Whole foods, 37
    Standard American/Australian Diet, 16
Digestion, aid to, 37, 40-41, 46, 48-49, 57, 58, 61, 64 (in pets, 69)
Don Tolman, 71
Dressings
    Avocado Aioli Dressing, recipe, 182
    Basic Vinaigrette, recipe, 182
    Coconut Citrus Vinaigrette, recipe, 178
    Creamy Coriander Dressing, recipe, 183
    Spicy Salad Dressing, recipe, 174
    Sweet Miso Dressing, recipe, 168
    Tahini Dressing, recipe, 182

E

Eczema, 12-13, 61-62
Energy boost, 26, 35, 46
Environmental toxins 60
Enzymes, 19, 37, 39, 41, 48, 49, 58
Essential Fatty Acids, 19
    Lauric acid, 19, 20, 27-28, 31, 48, 53, 62
    Short chain (SCFA), 19, 26, 32
    Medium chain (MCFA), 19, 28, 32, 33, 46, 47, 49, 62
    Long chain (LCFA) 19, 32, 46
Essential oils, 32, 42, 61
Exfoliant, 64

F

Falafels With Tahini Yoghurt, recipe, 136
Fats
    Chemistry of fats, 17

Diglycerides, 19
Monoglycerides, 19, 21
Polyunsaturated, 17-18, 19, 21, 55, 60, 66
Saturated, 17-19, 21, 22, 28, 32, 37, 39, 55
Trans fats, 16, 18, 42,
Triglycerides, 19, 20, 47
Unsaturated, 17, 55, 66
Fermented foods, 40-41, 57
Fife, Dr Bruce, 12, 34, 48, 56, 57, 58, 61, 66
Fish oils, 17, 21
Flax Oil Dressing, recipe, 162
Fructose, 24-26, 46
Fungus, 35, 61

G

Gallbladder disease, 19, 40, 46, 49, 61
Genetically modified (GMO), 41-42
Glucose, 24, 26, 46, 48, 50
Gluten, gluten-free, 41, 45
Glycaemic index, 24, 25, 26, 37
Grain-Free Vegetable Pizza, recipe, 140
Green Detox Soup, recipe, 124

H

Hair, 35, 42, 45, 54, 64-65
Hempseed Tabouli, recipe, 180
Honey, 25, 26
Hormones, 18, 35, 47, 54-55, 58

I

Ice-Cream,
Acai Berry Coconut Ice Cream, recipe, 214
Coconut Ice Cream, recipe, 204
Infant health, 20, 21, 49, 53
Inulin, 26

L

Labels, labeling, 18, 27, 31, 36, 41, 42
Lauric acid, 19, 20, 27-28, 31, 48, 53, 62
Lentils
    Coconut Lentil Curry With Cauliflower Rice, recipe, 134
    Lemon Lentil Soup, recipe, 120
    Spicy Lentil Salad, recipe, 174
Lip balm, 35, 45, 64
Liver, 18, 19, 24-25, 46-47, 49, 50, 55

M

Magnesium, sources of, 26, 40
Maple syrup, 26
Mental clarity, 35
MCT oil, 20, 31, 49, 50
Milks
Almond Milk, recipe, 108
Hempseed Milk, recipe, 108
Miso; Sweet Miso Dressing, recipe, 168
Moisturiser, 35, 61-62, 64
MSG – monosodium glutamate, 42

N

Nappy rash cream, 54
Nose bleeds, 45
Nut Cheeses
Easy Cashew Cheese, recipe, 114
Macadamia Cream Cheese, recipe 114
NutraSweet, 27

O

Obesity, 16, 18, 47, 49
Oleic acid (Omega-9), 20, 21
Oils Types
Almond, 19
Avocado, 19
Canola, 18, 19
Corn, 18, 19
Cottonseed, 18
Flaxseed, 22
Hempseed, 21
Macadamia, 19
Margarine, 18, 45, 60
Olive, 17, 18, 19, 22, 27, 33
Palm, 17, 18,19
Peanut, 19, 22
Vegetable, 17, 18, 19, 37, 42, 55
Sesame seed, 19
Soybean, 19
Walnut, 19
Wheat germ, 22
Omega-3, 20-22, 39
Omega-6, 20-22, 39
Omega-9, 20-22
Oral hygiene

Dental problems, root canals, 27, 58
Oil pulling, 27, 58
Teething, 54
Toothpaste, 64, recipe 226

P

Pancreatitis, 49
Pizza; Grain-Free Vegetable Pizza, recipe, 140
Pumpkin Soup, recipe, 120
Prostaglandins, 21

Q

Quinoa
Coconut Quinoa With Kale & Pesto, recipe, 138
Quinoa Herb Salad, recipe, 172

R

Raspberry Sauce, recipe, 204
Raw chocolate
Berry Coconut Chocolate, recipe, 186
Bounty Bars, recipe, 188
Cherry Choc Slice, recipe, 196
Chocolate Fruit Pie, recipe, 200
Chocolate Mousse, recipe, 192
Coconut Peppermint Slice, recipe, 190
Maca Macaroons, recipe, 188
Mocha Magic Bites, recipe, 194
Orange Chocolate Mousse Cake, recipe, 198
Raw Cacao & Coconut Fudge, recipe, 186
White Chocolate, recipe, 186
Raw desserts
Acai Berry Coconut Ice-Cream, recipe, 214
Avocado & Coconut Popsicles, recipe, 218
Berry Bliss Bars, recipe, 212
Choc Almond Bliss Balls, recipe, 216
Coconut & Lime Cheesecake, recipe, 206
Coconut Rough Bliss Balls, recipe, 216
Lemon & Coconut Nut-Free Slice, recipe, 210
Raw Apple Pie With Coconut Cream, recipe, 208
Raw Coconut Ice-Cream With Raspberry Sauce, recipe, 204
Raw food, 13, 22, 25, 27, 37, 57, 69
Raw meals
Raw Avocado & Cucumber Soup, recipe, 128

Raw Coconut Soup, recipe, 126
Raw Lasagna, recipe, 154
Raw Pad Thai With Kelp Noodles, recipe, 148
Raw Soft Tacos With Walnut Meat, recipe, 146
Raw Tom Yum Soup, recipe, 146
Raw Vegan Tuna Salad, recipe, 150
Raw Vegetable Patties, recipe, 152
Raw Zucchini Pasta With Basil Sauce, recipe, 144

Roasted Cauliflower With Coconut + Spice, recipe, 162
Roasted Eggplant Soup, recipe, 124
Roasted Vegetables In Coconut Magic Coconut Oil, recipe, 142

S

Salads
Coleslaw + Coconut Citrus Vinaigrette, recipe, 178
Greek Salad With Almond Feta, recipe, 170
Hemp Seed Tabouli, recipe, 180
Kale & Avocado Salad With Sweet Miso, recipe 168
Quinoa Herb Salad, recipe, 172
Spicy Lentil Salad, recipe, 174
Steamed Green Vegetable Salad, recipe, 176
Sex/ sexual function, 54-55, 67
Skin tissue damage, 60-62, 67
Skin wounds, 61
Soups
Carrot, Ginger & Sweet Potato Soup, recipe, 118
Creamy Tomato Basil Soup, recipe, 128
Green Detox Soup, recipe, 124
Lemon Lentil Soup, recipe, 120
Pumpkin Soup, recipe, 120
Raw Avocado & Cucumber Soup, recipe, 128
Raw Coconut Soup, recipe, 126
Raw Tom Yum Soup, recipe, 126
Roasted Eggplant Soup, recipe, 124
Thai Style Coconut & Vegetable Soup, recipe, 122
Soy products, 18, 19, 22, 40-41, 45, 47, 60
Stevia, 26
Stretch marks, 35, 53, 64
Stress relief, 35
Sucrose, 24, 26
Sugars
Cane, 24, 25, 27

Coconut sugar, 25-26, 45
Coconut nectar, 25-26, 37, 41, 45
Corn syrup, 24, 27
Equal, 27
Fructose, 24-26, 46
Glucose, 24, 26, 46, 48, 50
Honey, 25, 26
Maple syrup, 26
NutraSweet, 27
Stevia, 26
Sucrose, 24, 26
Sweet'N Low, 26
Sunscreen 65
Superfoods, 36, 37, 39, 44
Sustainability, 25, 28, 44
Sweet Miso Dressing, recipe, 168
Sweet potato - Coconut Crusted Sweet Potato Chips, recipe, 164

T

Tahini Dressing, recipe, 182
Tahini Yoghurt, recipe, 136
Teething, 54
Therese Kerr, 71
Thyroid support 40, (in pregnancy, 53), 54-55
Tomato Sauce, recipe, 164

V

Vaginal health, 67
Vegan Moussaka, recipe, 132
Vinaigrette, recipe, 182
Vitamins, 22, 26, 37, 41, 49, 53, 61

W

Weight loss, 19, 34, 47, 49, 64

Y

Yeast infections/candida, 54
Yoghurt
Cashew Yoghurt, recipe 112
Coconut Milk Yoghurt, recipe 112

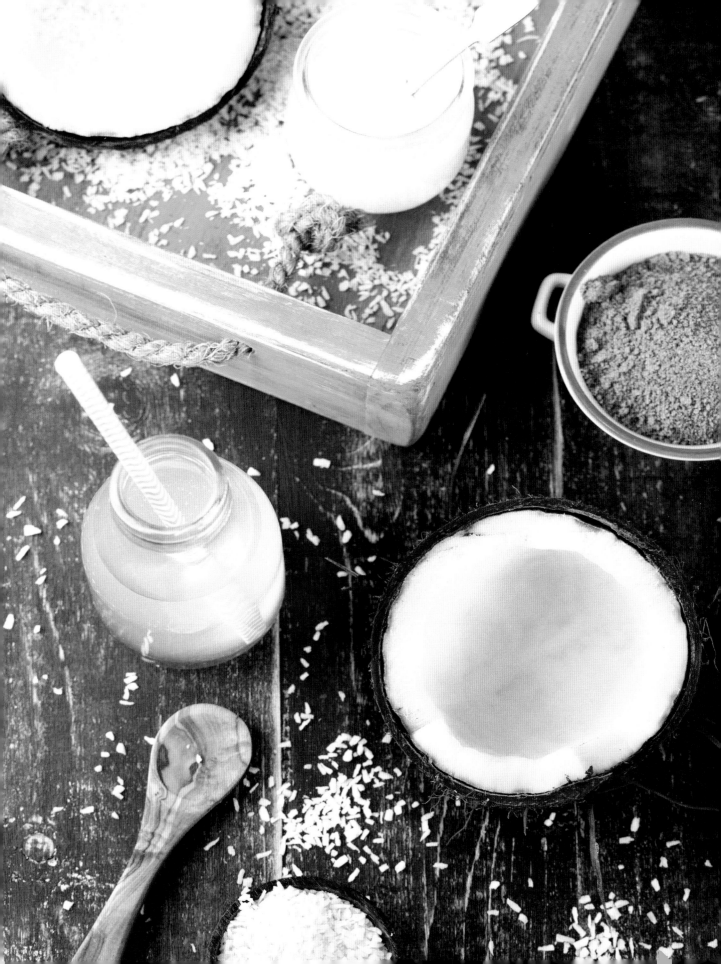

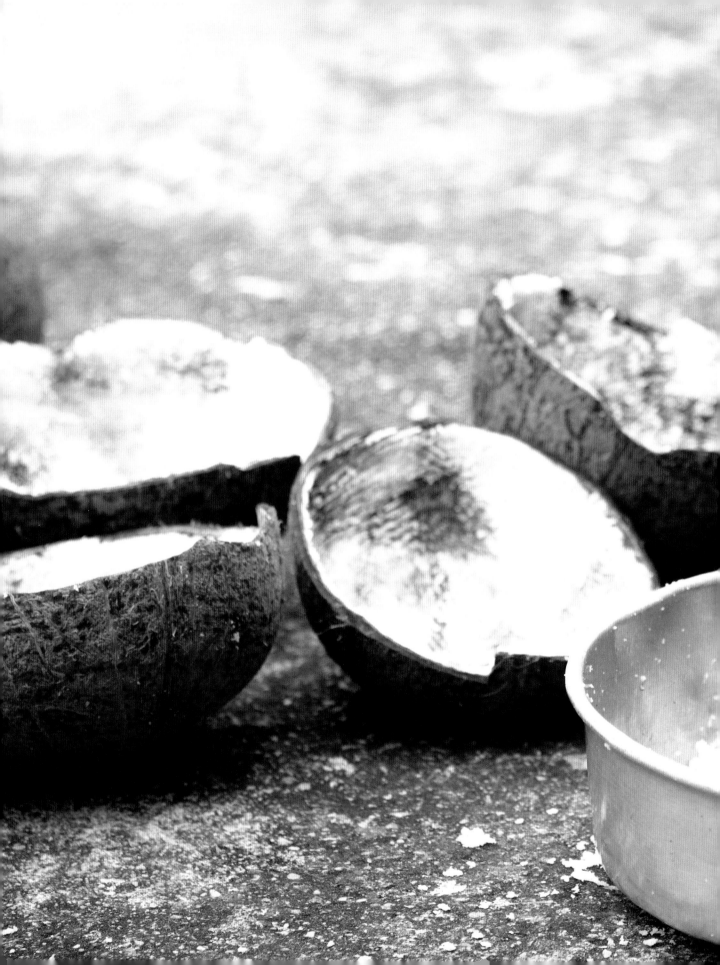

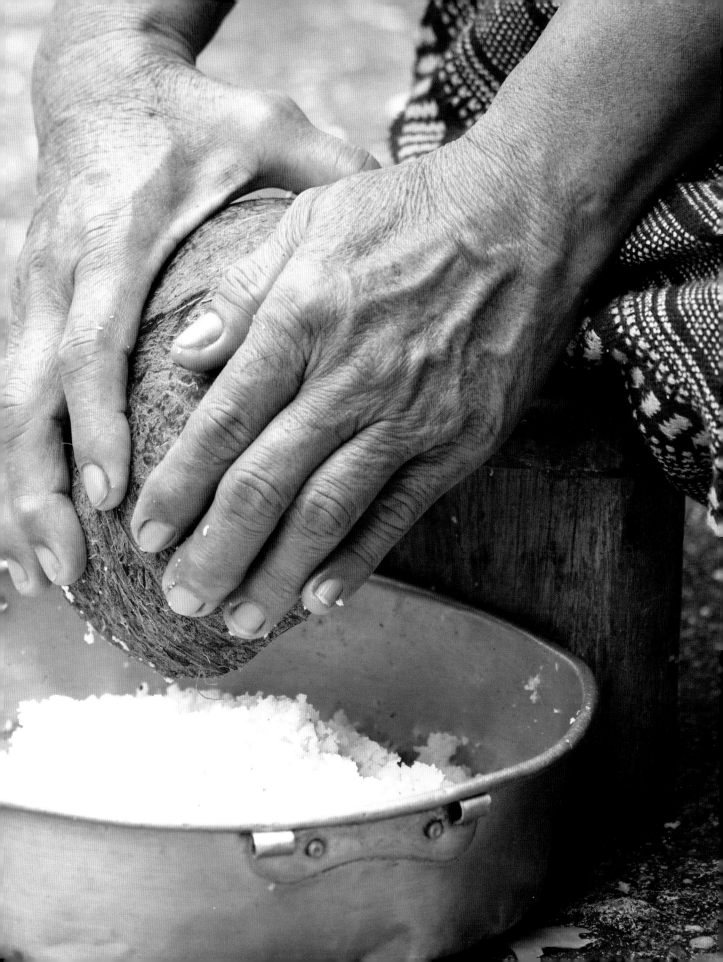

ACKNOWLEDGEMENTS

Thank you to everyone who has supported the Coconut Magic brand. Many of you have been with me since the start of my coconut oil journey, and many continue to join us along the way. I am grateful for your loyalty to our products and enthusiasm for what the Coconut Magic brand stands for. You make me want to get up each day and do more for our communities. Without you Coconut Magic would not exist, and this book could not have been possible.

My heartfelt gratitude goes to my husband, Andrew, who taste-tested every single one of my recipes and became my stamp of approval. From you came the encouragement and support I needed to see this through.

My gorgeous dog Mocha is a living example of how coconut oil can benefit pets, as she enters her senior years so gracefully.

My friends Sandy and John, who trusted me with financial backing in the early days of starting the business, when I had nothing but a crazy passion for Coconut Magic oil, and for their continued support to this day.

To Vance who visits us regularly and is always eager to taste-test recipes and offer compliments, insights and fresh ideas.

Former and current team members at Coconut Magic, who took part in the taste-testing, contributed their ideas and helped develop some of the recipes.

My friends Silvi and Nick, from Divine by Therese Kerr, for loaning us their amazing home, Serenity House in Casuarina Beach, for our photo shoots.

Our team in Thailand for continuing to make the most amazing coconut products, answering my ongoing questions, accommodating my frequent visits, and for patiently teaching me and showing me the production methods and farming of our Coconut Magic products. This has been the foundation for the beginning of my research and the entire coconut journey.

And of course the hands-on team of Gaynor, Vanessa, Isabella and Suze; you worked by my side many long hours, sometimes day and night, with focus and determination to help make it all happen.

ABOUT THE AUTHOR

Jenni Madison adopted the healthy coconut lifestyle when she first discovered coconut oil while living and working in Thailand, and used it to resolve her chronic digestive and skin-related issues.

But she found that not all coconut oils are the same. After extensive research she discovered that quality depends on the time of harvesting, the extraction process and even how the oil is packaged and delivered. Coconut oil had become her passion!

Returning to Australia, Jenni founded Coconut Magic, a fair-trade company that distributes premium quality coconut oil, coconut products and raw energy bars.

This book comes from a passion and a desire to share the magic of coconuts for healing and as the basis of a healthy lifestyle rich in wholefoods, plant-based foods and superfoods.

The mission of *The Healthy Coconut* is simple: to share nutrition tips and recipes that allow you to introduce the magic of coconut into your daily lifestyle.

Jenni Madison lives in Kingscliff, NSW, Australia with her husband Andrew, and their German Shepherd and coconut-loving dog, Mocha. Andrew recently joined Coconut Magic as co-owner and Manger of Operations. Together they enjoy a healthy coconut, beach-side lifestyle.

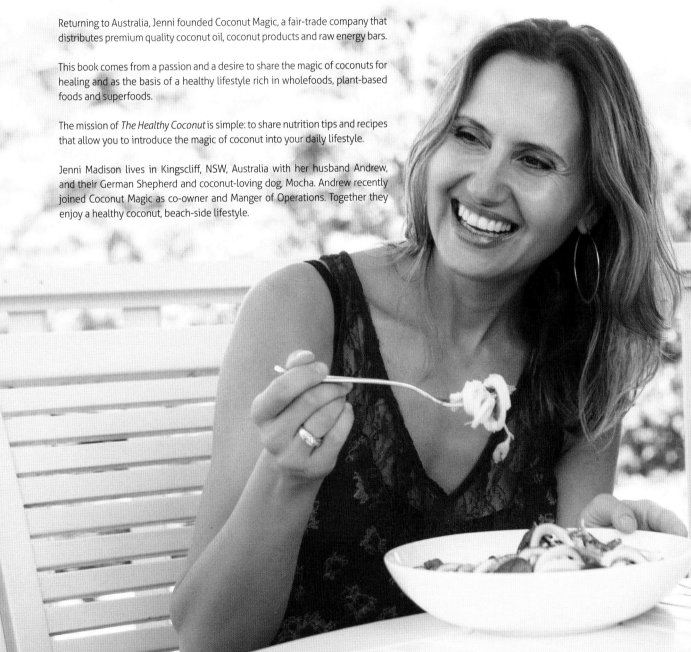

A Rockpool book
PO Box 252
Summer Hill, NSW 2130
Australia

www.rockpoolpublishing.com.au
www.facebook.com/RockpoolPublishing

This edition published in 2016

First published in 2015 by Earth Born Publishing
www.coconutmagic.com

Copyright © Jenni Madison, 2015
Photography © Earth Born Publishing

A copy of this publication can be found in the National Library of Australia.

ISBN 978-1-925429-07-7

DISCLAIMER: This book is intended to serve as an introduction to healthy lifestyle changes. Information contained in this book is based on the experience and research of the author. It should not be treated as a definitive guide, nor should it be considered to cover every area of concern, or be regarded as legal or medical advice. Readers should always consult an appropriate health professional on matters relating to their well-being. Neither the author nor the publisher and their distributors can be held responsible for any loss, claim or action that may arise from reliance on the information contained in this book. See your health practitioner for a full medical check-up before embarking on any new diet.

Edited by Gaynor Foster
Art Director/Designer by Vanessa Russell
Photography by Suze McLeod
Food Styling by Vanessa Russell
Photography Location Serenity House
All other images sourced from Shutterstock and Dollarphotos.
Printed in China

If you enjoyed The Healthy Coconut and want to know more:
Visit **www.coconutmagic.com**
For advice, tips, latest updates, recipes and more...
Find Jenni Madison on Facebook on **www.facebook.com/coconutmagic**
or coconut recipes on Instagram: **www.instagram.com/coconutmagic**